THE MEDICO-LEGAL BACK:
AN ILLUSTRATED GUIDE

THE MEDICO-LEGAL BACK: AN ILLUSTRATED GUIDE

Robert A Dickson

MA, MB, ChM, FRCS, FRCSE, DSc
Professor of Orthopaedic Surgery, University of Leeds
Consultant Orthopaedic Spine Surgeon, St James's University
Hospital and the Leeds General Infirmary
Director, Yorkshire Regional Complex Spine Treatment Centre
Director, University of Leeds Centre for Spinal Research
Past President, British Scoliosis Society

W Paul Butt

MD, FRCP(C), FRCR
Senior Consultant, Musculo-skeletal and Spine Radiologist
St James's University Hospital and the Leeds General Infirmary
Senior Clinical Lecturer, Orthopaedic Radiology, University of Leeds
Lately Member of Council, Royal College of Radiologists
Past President, British Society of Skeletal Radiologists

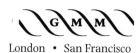

London • San Francisco

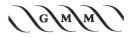

© 2004

Greenwich Medical Media Limited
4th Floor, 137 Euston Road,
London
NW1 2AA

870 Market Street, Ste 720
San Francisco
CA 94109, USA

ISBN 1 84110 167 2

First Published 2004

A catalogue record for this book is available from the British Library.

www.greenwich-medical.co.uk

Typeset by Charon Tec Pvt. Ltd, Chennai, India

Printed in the UK by The Cromwell Press

CONTENTS

FOREWORD

This is a practitioner's book. It is an illustrated guide rather than a textbook, and it will be of immense value in the medico-legal world. How I wish that it had been available during my 40 years of grappling with claims for negligence for back injuries both at the Bar and on the Bench. It would have saved many hours of searching for suitable background information and explanation on an area of the body which is complex and often produces problems that are so difficult to define and nail down that they produce differing expert opinions.

The paramount virtue of this book is that the text is expressed with a clarity which makes it easy to read and readily understandable. Of particular help are the many analogies, which are drawn between anatomical technicalities and movements, situations and incidents, which are part of everyday life. To clarify matters even further, there are abundant illustrations and drawings to augment the text and these help the reader to visualise the problems facing the court. It will be of great assistance to the busy lawyer, especially those who come into a case at a very late stage and have to prepare it under the pressure of time. I suspect that it will be of equal value to orthopaedic and neurosurgeons who are building up their medico-legal experience.

The authors are eminently qualified to produce a book of this kind, as they have added their combined extensive medico-legal experience to their already impressive academic records. Robert Dickson is Professor of Orthopaedic Surgery at the University of Leeds and a Consultant Orthopaedic Surgeon at St James's University Hospital and The Leeds General Infirmary. Paul Butt is the Senior Consultant Musculo-skeletal and Spine Radiologist at St James's University Hospital and The Leeds General Infirmary, and Senior Lecturer in Orthopaedic Radiology at the University of Leeds. They have worked in collaboration for almost a quarter of a century, during which time they have built up an international reputation for the Yorkshire Regional Centre for Spinal Surgery in the fields of children's spinal problems and adult reconstructive spinal work. They have also developed an academic spinal centre where expert knowledge of the relevant applied sciences is blended with the authors' knowledge of medical science.

I am sure that this book will quickly become a valued and trusted friend to all those who have the need to refer to it.

His Honour Donald Herrod Q.C.
January 2004

PREFACE

A quarter of a century ago one of us (WPB) arrived as a Consultant Radiologist with a particular interest in the musculo-skeletal system at St James's University Hospital in Leeds. Shortly thereafter, the other (RAD) took up the position of Professor of Orthopaedic Surgery in the same institution and from then on we have worked on a daily basis seeking to provide an optimal clinical service for patients in the Yorkshire region, and beyond, who have spinal problems. It became abundantly clear that *imaging* (all forms of X-rays and scans) was an essential partner to safe, sensible, well-intentioned spinal surgery with a minimal complication rate. Thus the spinal surgeon and the spinal radiologist must work together to produce clinical work of the highest quality. Back then, we instituted a regular weekly audit meeting (long before audit was ever envisaged) whereby all patients operated upon the following week were assessed clinically and radiologically by the spinal team (spinal surgeons, nurses, radiologists etc). This practice of course continues today although, mercifully, there is more than one spinal surgeon and one radiologist!

Because we emphasise in this text that, apart from red flag problems such as cancer, scanning in particular has to be surgically-directed, then the marrying up of clinical features with scan appearances is an absolutely essential pre-requisite before surgical intervention. In addition, our regional complex spinal unit receives at least one, and often more, patients a day with something like secondary cancer of the spine causing spinal cord compression, a spinal fracture or tuberculosis of the spine which requires surgical intervention. It would be unheard of in our Unit for such imaging not to be performed by one of our spinal radiologists and for the appearances not to be thoroughly discussed between surgeon or radiologist prior to surgical intervention. We provide that level of clinical service and although proud of it would not deem any other level of practice acceptable.

We also believe very strongly that expert witnesses should have very considerable experience in the clinical conditions which they seek to report upon. For the past decade and a half RAD has been involved solely in spinal matters and would therefore not put himself forward as an expert witness in, say, matters to do with the foot and ankle or the shoulder. Similarly WPB, a trained and expert musculo-skeletal radiologist would not put himself forward as an expert in soft parts. Both of us may know a fair amount about sub-specialties outside our own clinical activity but we would not go forward to the Courts of this land as an expert witness.

Because the musculo-skeletal system, and the spine in particular, depends so much upon imaging, then to provide an expert opinion in Court more than often involves a combination of spinal surgical and spinal radiological opinion. We have therefore worked very closely together for more than a decade in medico-legal work and we have always addressed the Court with our opinions long before the more recent reforms of Lord Woolf. We would provide exactly the same report, word for word, whether instructed by Claimants or Defendants and we staunchly support Lord Woolf's initiatives. Doctors must appear "for themselves".

Where there is a paucity of information underpinning a clinical or radiological matter there certainly is opportunity for differing opinions. The last several decades have seen an exponential wealth of published material that provides, in most circumstances, a very sound factual basis underscoring an expert's opinion. This is called "evidence-based medicine" and we have sought in this short text to produce, albeit in a fairly elementary and pictorial way, what we consider the essential facts from which an opinion can be drawn.

We have written this text in the form of an illustrated guide particularly with our legal colleagues in mind. More often than not when we produce reports or go to Court to be questioned about them, we are asked for pictorial evidence to assist Solicitors, Counsel and the Judiciary. That is therefore what we have done in this text and if we have used too simple analogies such as "the vertebra in cross-section being like a house with the body being the house itself and the posterior arch being the roof with the spinal clockwork in the attic" then we offer our apologies to those who already know their spinal anatomy. For those who don't, we hope that such analogies, and others to everyday life, will prove helpful.

We have tried to as far as possible provide evidence rather than opinion but if on occasion opinion does seem to come through then it is one that is held on the basis of good evidence and also one that is quite capable of being updated according to whatever new and reliable information appears in our journals or through clinical experience. It is thus a living text. Perhaps in ten years time when the second edition is published, if indeed there is a second edition, the evidence-base might have changed but this text presents how it is now and for the foreseeable future.

We have covered all areas of spinal surgery from degenerative disc disease through to spinal deformities in children because all, in their own way, do have significant medico-legal ramifications. However because degenerative spine disease and the interaction between back pain and litigation do have an important place medico-legally in this country, and indeed many others, we have gone into these matters in a bit more detail supplying relevant references so that interested readers might wish to take their knowledge further.

We hope that lawyers involved with medico-legal spinal work will find value from the text and the many illustrations, and we would also hope that some young orthopaedic or neurosurgical spinal surgeons, setting out on their medico-legal careers, might also derive some benefit. We confirm that we are entirely interactive and would welcome any feedback from any source.

Robert A Dickson (RAD)
W Paul Butt (WPB)
2004

ACKNOWLEDGEMENTS

In the drafting of this text we were very keen to seek the help and advice from a range of legal opinion and a number of orthopaedic surgeons with an interest in spinal surgery. We sent the first draft to an experienced circuit Judge, to Senior Counsel, to a big firm of lawyers working for Plaintiffs and a big firm of lawyers working for Defendants. We are grateful for all their helpful comments which have been incorporated in the text. As Professor Gordon Waddell has been such a key player in this field, we also invited him to inspect and comment on our first draft which he kindly did and we then went back and forth until we felt that his position had been properly described.

David Limb and Peter Millner, two young and brainy orthopaedic surgeons in Leeds, were kind enough to read the final draft and validate it with their approval.

Mrs Helen Radcliffe (RAD's secretary) typed and word-processed the text, Mr David Sharples (our orthopaedic technician) assisted greatly in the production of the illustrations and Mr Paul Fleming and his staff in the Medical Illustration Department of St James's Hospital, Leeds were also of great assistance. We thank them all.

Some Useful Words

Words are important in both medicine and law. Many medical terms come from either Latin or Greek and quite a lot of them refer to the *anatomy* (structure) of the body. Although whole bodies are no longer dissected as part of the undergraduate medical course, only the odd part thereof, because factual over-load dictates that there is not enough time, anatomy still forms an essential part of the language of medicine. We shall come to some of the more awkward, perhaps confusing, words (such as *spondylosis*, *spondylitis*, *spondylolysis* and *spondylolisthesis*) in due course in their relevant sections but it may be useful to run over a few directional/locational terms now. *Spondyl* means spine and then you add on what is wrong with it.

- Spondylosis – degenerative (wear and tear) arthritis (osis: degeneration)
- Spondylitis – inflammatory arthritis (itis: inflammation)
- Spondylolysis – stress fracture at bottom of spine (lysis: stress fracture)
- Spondylolisthesis – slippage forward of one vertebra on another (olisthesis: slippage)

Just as any body in space can be described in terms of its three fundamental planes so we refer to the human body's three *planes* (flat surfaces) (Fig. 1.1). If the body is sliced from front to back into right and left halves, this is the *sagittal* plane from the

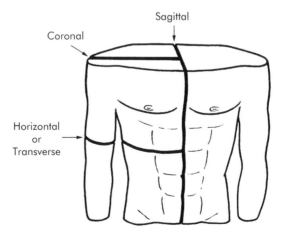

Fig. 1.1   The three planes of the body.

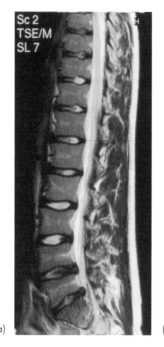

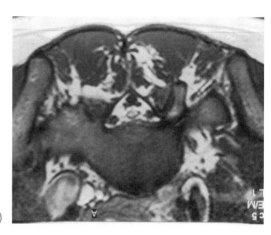

(a)   (b)

Fig. 1.2   MRI scan slices of the spine. (a) Sagittal slice or sideways look at the spine. (b) Axial slice or cross-sectional look at the spine.

Latin for arrow (which was presumably thought to attack you purely in this direction). If the body is sliced side to side into front and back halves, this is referred to as the *frontal* or *coronal* (like a crown) plane; and if the body is sliced in cross section, this is referred to as the *transverse, horizontal* or *axial* plane. It is important to remember these planes – sagittal, coronal and transverse – as this is how, for instance, magnetic resonance imaging (MRI) scans are described and interpreted (Fig. 1.2).

The front of the body is referred to as *anterior* or *ventral* and the back as *posterior* or *dorsal* and if one structure is in front of another it is ventral or anterior to it, and, if it is behind it, it is dorsal or posterior (Fig. 1.3). Therefore, the sternum (breastbone) is anterior to the spine, which in turn is posterior to the sternum. Meanwhile, if something is higher in the body than another it is referred to as *superior* or *cranial* (towards the head). If it is lower it is *inferior* or *caudal* (towards the tail). Thus, the brain is superior to the heart, while the legs are inferior to the back. Fairly obviously, if something is on the outside it is *external* and on the inside *internal*, and if it is on the surface it

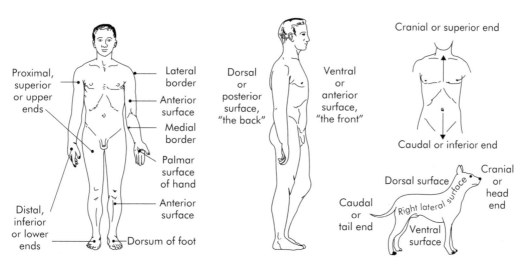

Fig. 1.3   Terms of relationship and comparison. From Grant JCB, Basmajian JV (1965). Grant's Method of Anatomy. Seventh Edition. E & S Livingstone. Edinburgh & London.

is *superficial* and if it is inside it is *deep*. Similarly, if something is closer to the midline it is *medial* and if it is further away it is *lateral*.

These terms are referable to a body standing, face forward, with palms forward. The little finger is, therefore, the most medial digit and the thumb the most lateral. A body lying face up is *supine* and face down is *prone*. Something closer to the centre is *proximal* and something further away is *distal*. The shoulder is, therefore, proximal to the elbow while the wrist is distal to the elbow.

As regards movements, when one leans forward to touch one's toes the spine is *flexed* and when one leans backward the spine *extends*. It can also bend to the right or left, *lateral* flexion (trying to push one's fingers down one's thighs), and *rotate* (twisting the spine so that one's head faces to the right or left). Thus, flexion and extension, lateral flexion and rotation are commonly used terms.

It is more easy to define terms than to use them in the clinical setting in that a patient with a serious spinal deformity might require their spinal joints to be fused from the neck down to the pelvis but they can, of course, touch their toes because their hip joints are normal. In other words, the entire movement is produced by the hip joints with the spine being completely stiff and this is why an important part of the examination of a patient is to watch where the movement is occurring rather than merely registering its extent. Thus, for instance, measuring fingertip to ground distance as an index of the amount of forward flexion, or for that matter less precisely recording spinal flexion in fractions of normal (e.g. half-normal or three-quarters normal), only crudely describes the range of motion unless it is observed that it is the spine itself which is flexing rather than the nearby articulations.

- Anterior – in front
- Posterior – behind
- Superior – above
- Inferior – below
- External – outside
- Internal – inside
- Superficial – near the surface
- Deep – underneath
- Medial – nearer the midline
- Lateral – further from the midline
- Supine – lying on one's back
- Prone – lying on one's front
- Flexion – bending forward
- Extension – bending backward
- Rotation – twisting

We shall do our best to explain the many other words and terms as and when we come to them.

Anatomy of the Spine

Anatomy means structure and the skeleton is made up of hard parts and soft parts. *Bones* are the supporting framework and they meet and move at *joints*. Bones also act as levers and are moved by *muscles*, which are sometimes attached directly to a bone or via a *tendon* (piece of stringy gristle). Muscles contract when signalled by electrical impulses supplied from *nerves*, which originate from the brain and spinal cord (*the central nervous system*) and branch out therefrom to their destinations (*the peripheral nervous system*). All this is kept alive by *blood*, which brings oxygen for movement and metabolism, and takes away the resultant waste products.

Bone consists of a framework of *fibrous* tissue (rather like a tendon) but with added calcium and phosphate salts. The fibrous component is made of a protein called *collagen* and gives bone its toughness, while the *mineral salts* give it its hardness and make bone visible on X-rays. Too little collagen (bone matrix) is called *osteoporosis* or brittle bone disease, and not enough mineral salts is called *osteomalacia* in adults and *rickets* in children (Fig. 2.1).

- Osteoporosis – not enough bone matrix
- Osteomalacia – not enough calcium salts

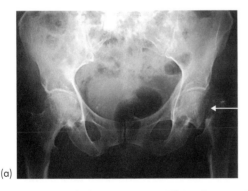 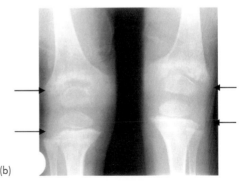

(a)   (b)

Fig. 2.1 (a) *Osteoporosis*. This picture of the pelvis shows very thin bone in the top of the thigh bones and on the left side (arrowed) is a fracture of the neck of the femur, which is a "pathological" fracture caused by a significant reduction in bone density. This is a very common fracture in the elderly and we shall see more and more of these as the elderly live longer and longer. (b) *Rickets*. There is widening, deformity and demineralisation of the growth plates on each side of the knee (arrowed). Compare this with the normal radiographic appearance (Fig. 2.4).

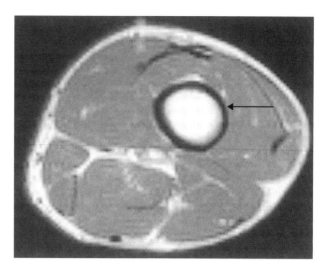

Fig. 2.2 MRI cross section of the thigh showing the bone, the femur (arrowed), in the middle, surrounded by muscles. Note that the bone is hollow and this is the diaphysis or mid-portion of the femur. The outer cortex which is black is of such strength that no bone is required inside.

Bone is either hard like ivory (*cortical bone*) or spongy like a honey-comb (*cancellous bone*). Cortical bone is on the outside and can-cellous bone on the inside. Sometimes, there is no cancellous bone at all inside, rather the inside is filled with no more than marrow, since a tubular rather than a solid cross section does not significantly reduce the strength of a bone (Fig. 2.2). This is because the contribution to the strength of the construct is very much greater the further from the centre; indeed it is pro-portional to the *square* of the distance from the middle of the bone (engineers call this the *second moment of area* or the *area moment of inertia* and rely a lot on materials with a tubular configuration). The advantages in turn for this are a marked reduction in body weight (otherwise we would be relatively immobile monsters) and that the inside of the bone can be used for other purposes, for example, to make blood cells and to store minerals.

The ivory cortical bone is very radio-dense and looks very white on X-rays (but black on MRIs). A tumour can completely occupy the marrow cavity inside without being recognised on X-rays provided that the surrounding cortical bone has not been eaten away (Fig. 2.3). Reciprocally, if a tumour in a bone

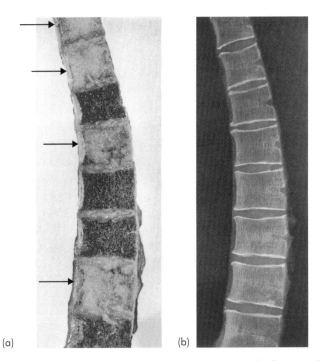

(a)   (b)

Fig. 2.3 This is the spine of a patient who died of secondary cancer. The spine was removed at autopsy and sectioned down the middle. (a) The specimen itself; (b) the specimen X-rayed. Several of the vertebrae have been replaced by white tumour (arrows) and indeed this patient succumbed from secondary cancer all over the body including the spine. Despite these gross appearances, the X-ray of the specimen (b) is entirely normal and this is because unless the outer cortical rim of the vertebra is destroyed by tumour, then the X-ray appearances will be entirely normal. Amazing perhaps, but it is true.

can be seen on X-ray it means that it has eroded cortical bone. Similarly, because cortical bone is so compact, osteoporosis cannot be recognised on an X-ray until at least 50% of the density of the bone has been lost. X-rays are undoubtedly invaluable in assessing the skeleton but implicit in any visible changes are that they are rather crude indices of disease or disorder – hence the evolution of more sensitive imaging techniques, such as *scanning*.

Bones are classified according to shape and, thus, the bone of the thigh (the *femur*) and that of the arm (the *humerus*) are *long bones*, while those of the *skull* and *shoulder blade* are *flat bones*. It might be thought that *vertebrae* being short in height are flat bones but they are in fact mini-long bones. Incidentally, arms and legs are very often incorrectly or at best loosely used words. Anatomically, the *arm* is between the shoulder and elbow, while the *leg* is between the knee and the ankle. Between the hip and the knee is the *thigh* and between the elbow and the wrist is the *forearm*. Meanwhile, the limb from hip downwards is referred to as the *lower limb* or *lower extremity*, and from shoulder downwards the *upper limb or upper extremity*. Thus, to say that the femur is not in the leg may sound slightly peculiar but is anatomically correct (it is in the thigh) and, therefore, in these circumstances it is better to use the term lower extremity.

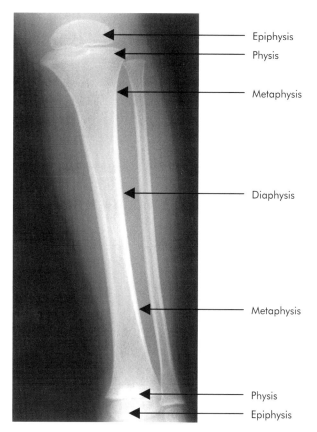

Epiphysis

Physis

Metaphysis

Diaphysis

Metaphysis

Physis

Epiphysis

Fig. 2.4 This is an AP X-ray of the tibia and fibula of a growing child to show the different anatomical areas with their respective names (compare to clarity of the physes with those in rickets [Fig. 2.1b]).

Bones grow at each end, or rather slightly below the top and slightly above the bottom, where there are special growth zones called *physes* (Fig. 2.4). At the ends of the growing bone beyond the physes are the *epiphyses*, while on the shaft side this area is called the *metaphysis* and the mid-shaft area, the *diaphysis*. Physes can be seen as radio-lucent lines on X-rays until maturity is reached, which is about 15 years in girls and 17 years in boys but, interestingly, spinal maturity is not reached until the early 20s. Bones are living organs and if fractured they have the ability to repair. In the young, and immature, repair may proceed all the way to normality as the original shape is restored but adults do not have the same *remodelling* capacity and, thus, X-rays after fractures in adults commonly show thickening, or a change in direction, length or alignment as a permanent reminder of injury.

While old injuries are not visible on X-rays taken of children, fresh injuries are and it may take 6 months or more for a long bone fracture in a child to remodel completely. Fractures look different on X-rays at different stages in their healing and this facilitates that tragic diagnosis of *child abuse* (non-accidental injury, NAI) (Fig. 2.5). Thus, several fractures dating from different times, as well as particular fracture sites or patterns, such as the back of the ribs, a fractured femur or tibia before the age of walking, and a transverse fracture direction in the walker may suggest NAI.

Ligaments (fibrous bands which protect joints) and muscles also have the ability to repair but no such facility was given to the *intervertebral disc*. Our *creator* was an accomplished biologist and engineer and, accordingly, provided very effective shock-absorbing mechanisms to protect the intervertebral disc. The idea that you can slip a disc bending or twisting or sneezing is as ludicrous as it is unchristian.

Bones meet together at *joints* and here the bones are separated from each other by *cartilage*, which is gristly, tough and resilient, rather like bone without its mineral salts. Not surprisingly, the major constituent of cartilage is collagen, just like bone. It is this cartilage layer that undergoes *degeneration* and gradually thins (wears) in *osteoarthritis* (Fig. 2.6).

Where joints have big ranges of movement, the ends of the bone are covered with a thin layer of white shiny cartilage

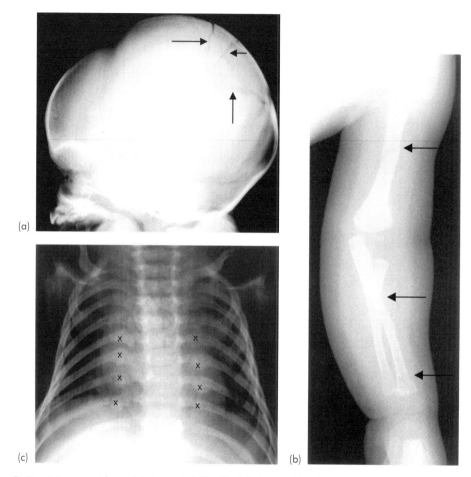

Fig. 2.5 *Non-accidental injury.* (a) Skull. (b) Arm. (c) Chest of the unfortunate infant who did not survive. The skull is fractured (arrows), there are three fractures in the same arm (arrows), and there are healing fractures at the back of the ribs (crosses) all in the same child.

referred to as *hyaline* cartilage. This can be seen, for example, at the end of a chicken drumstick. If, following injury, the bone ends part company completely, this is called *dislocation*; if they displace but not completely, this is called *subluxation*. With spinal injuries such displacement can have catastrophic consequences as the nearby spinal cord can be damaged resulting in paralysis (Fig. 2.7).

Hyaline cartilage is less tough and less strong than another type of cartilage, called *fibrocartilage*, which is very similar to the structure of a ligament. In the spine fibrocartilage occurs in

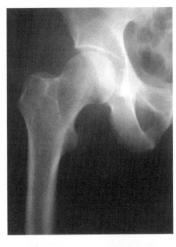

(a)

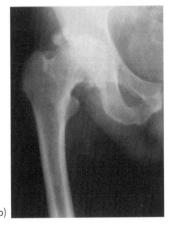

(b)

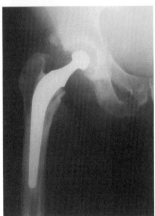

(c)

Fig. 2.6 (a) AP X-ray of a normal hip joint. Observe the gap between the ball (femoral head) and the socket (acetabulum). This is filled with articular cartilage (½ cm of gristle). (b) AP X-ray of a hip with severe degenerative arthritis. There isn't any joint space – in other words the articular cartilage has worn away completely. As a result the bone on each side has thickened because of increased stresses and there is marginal new bone formation (osteophytes). (Patient of Mr David Macdonald). (c) AP X-ray following a Charnley total hip replacement.

intervertebral discs, and makes the disc by far the strongest structure in the human spine.

- Ligaments – stabilise joints
- Tendons – attach muscles to bone
- Cartilage – gristle where bones make joints

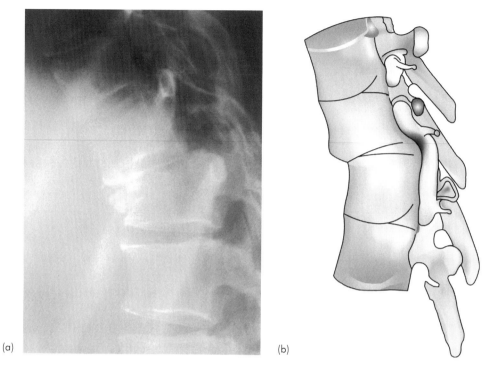

(a)   (b)

Fig. 2.7   (a) Lateral radiograph of a nasty fracture–dislocation showing forward displacement of the vertebra above on the one below. (b) Drawing of the same.

Between two adjacent vertebrae, there are in fact three different types of joints. Therefore, while we may talk loosely of an *intervertebral joint* between two adjacent vertebrae, each so-called intervertebral joint consists of three different parts, which are in fact three anatomically discrete types of joint. On the top and bottom flat surfaces of each vertebra, there is a thin layer of hyaline cartilage and these are separated by a much thicker layer of fibrocartilage, which has evolved over millennia into the intervertebral disc with the fibrocartilaginous surrounding *annulus* and the central gelatinous *nucleus* (Fig. 2.8). This joint configuration of bone, hyaline cartilage, fibrocartilage, hyaline cartilage and bone, is referred to as a *symphysis* and a similar configuration occurs at the front of the pelvis where the two pubic bones come together. Then every joint has a surrounding fibrous *capsule*. This capsule does not amount to much in the shoulder joint, for example, which has such a huge range of motion in all directions. However, symphyses have immensely strong capsules and where the fibrous capsule is particularly strong or thickened, or runs in a particular

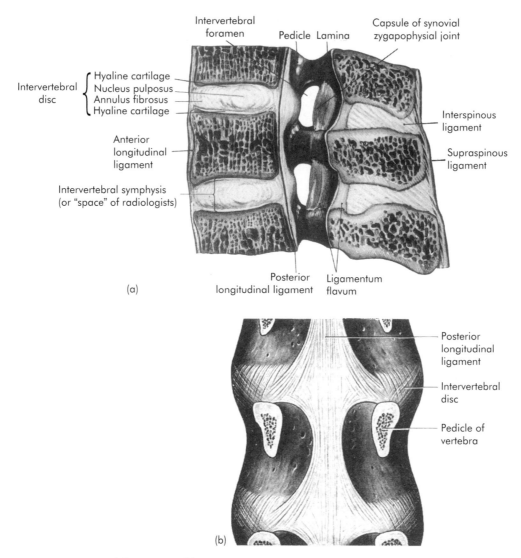

Fig. 2.8 *Some of the spine's fibrous tissue structures.* (a) Part of a spine split in the sagittal plane showing the vertebral bodies and intervening discs on the left, the spinal canal where the nerves are in the middle, and the spinous processes with the intervening interspinous ligaments in between on the right. Note the number of ligamentous structures which protect the spine starting at the front – anterior longitudinal ligament, annulus fibrosus, posterior longitudinal ligament, ligamentum flavum, capsule of synovial joint, interspinous ligament, supraspinous ligament (you do not need to remember their names!). (b) Looking into the front of the spinal canal from the back (i.e. in the frontal plane) with the roof of the house removed as well as the spinal cord. The posterior longitudinal ligament and the annulus of the intervertebral disc are seen to be interwoven together with broad expansions of the posterior longitudinal ligament at disc level – an immensely strong construct. From Gray's Anatomy (1989). Eds Williams PL, Warwick R, Dyson M, Bannister LH. Thirty-Seventh Edition. Churchill Livingstone. Edinburgh & London.

direction, it is referred to as a ligament. The intervertebral discs are protected by ligaments of enormous strength. The notion that discs can be affected by anything other than, say, a very high-speed road-traffic accident or a fall from a great height is, therefore, quite untenable.

Then at the back of the bony spine, where the bony arches meet on each side, the *articular processes* form a *synovial* joint similar to limb joints (Fig. 2.9). Finally, the bony prominences sticking out from the back and side of the spine (the *spinous* and *transverse processes*) are joined by strong fibrous tissue ligaments and this joint configuration is referred to as a *syndesmosis*.

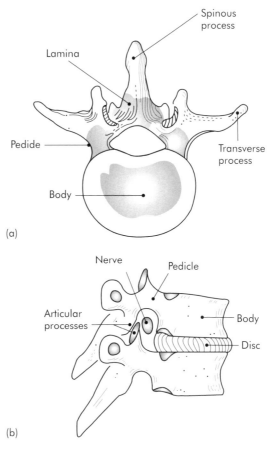

Fig. 2.9   (a) Transverse view and (b) lateral view of a lumbar vertebra. From Grant JCB, Basmajian JV (1965). Grant's Method of Anatomy. Seventh Edition. E & S Livingstone. Edinburgh & London.

These intervertebral joint complexes have evolved to allow the human spine to optimally carry out its mechanical functions with a considerable degree of in-built safety, which would entirely accord with its requirement to protect the spinal cord and its branches from the base of the skull down to the pelvis.

Joints facilitate movement and for this to occur in a controlled fashion requires muscular activity. Muscles are specialised forms of connective tissue with fibres, which can contract, approximate bones, and produce joint movements. Muscles are named after the Latin word for a mouse (*musculus*), perhaps somewhat surprisingly, but on reflection the mouse and its tail do nicely represent the two essential parts of a skeletal muscle – the lean muscle itself being the mouse's body and the fibrous tendon of insertion into bone being the mouse's tail. Tendons are incredibly strong and for this reason can be of very small calibre in relation to the muscle belly itself. With advancing age some tendons, for example the Achilles tendon, can spontaneously degenerate and lose strength, but otherwise tendons are so immensely strong that it is the rule that they pull off a piece of bone at their attachment rather than tear through the tendon substance itself.

When we are born, our spine describes a gentle C-shape from top to bottom and with the head on top resembles a comma. As the child begins to develop head control and look about, the back of the neck becomes hollow and then when the child starts to walk and be upright a comparable hollow develops in the lower part of the spine behind the abdomen. Thus, after the first year of life, the spine in lateral (sideways) profile is gently S-shaped being hollow (*lordosis*) behind the *cervical* (neck) and *lumbar* (low back) regions and being rounded or convex backwards (*kyphosis*) in the *thoracic* or chest part of the spine and down in the lower part of the spine referred to as the *sacro-coccygeal* region (Fig. 2.10). The kyphoses allow maximum volume for the chest and pelvic organs in front of them, while the contents of these areas are further protected by the presence of the ribs and bony pelvis, respectively. The chest and pelvis portions of the spine, therefore, serve a different function from the neck and lumbar spine, do not permit as much movement and, therefore, do not require powerful muscles to support them. By contrast, the cervical and lumbar lordoses are the two areas of the spine with maximum movement and they are controlled

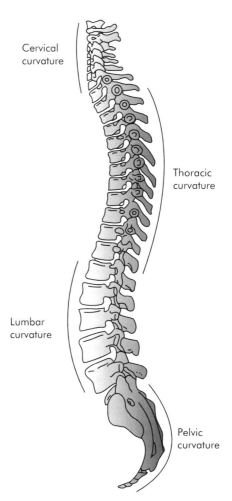

Cervical
curvature

Thoracic
curvature

Lumbar
curvature

Pelvic
curvature

Fig. 2.10   The spine is naturally curved in the sagittal plane with thoracic and sacro-coccygeal kyphoses and cervical and lumbar lordoses. The thoraco-lumbar spine is made up of twelve thoracic and five lumbar vertebrae. From Gray's Anatomy (1989). Eds Williams PL, Warwick R, Dyson M, Bannister LH. Thirty-Seventh Edition. Churchill Livingstone. Edinburgh & London.

by particularly powerful muscular and ligamentous structures behind them. The muscles running down the back of the spine are collectively referred to as the *erector spinae*, while the ligaments making up the cervical and lumbar joints are the strongest in the human body. It is the erector spinae musculoligamentous system, which maintains the erect posture (not surprisingly) in just the same way that guy ropes hold up tent poles and masts are held up by rigging. This is nicely exemplified by the fact that a skeleton prepared without this muscle mass promptly collapses under a weight of a mere 2 kg (the weight of one adult head). Such spinal collapse would produce a sideways bend (*scoliosis*).

- Kyphosis – round back
- Lordosis – hollow back
- Scoliosis – sideways bend

While the erector spinae does clearly have a major role in maintaining the erect position, it also has a very important role in spinal flexion. The good Lord (God, not my Lord) realised it would be very mechanically disadvantageous if the muscles that flex the spine were attached very close to the front of the spine and, therefore, he put the spinal flexors in the front of the abdominal wall to give them a decent lever arm. However, when one flexes fully forward to touch one's toes the abdominal musculature does not in fact contract and this can be verified by carrying out electromyography (EMG) during spinal flexion with needles inserted into the abdominal muscles which record no electrical activity whatever. This is because spinal flexion is accomplished by the posterior erector spinae muscle mass paying out rather as a pulley is lowered from the ceiling by paying out the rope.

Thus, to exercise one's abdominal musculature and to get rid of the middle-age spread, a very inefficient way of trying to do this would be to stand and repetitively touch one's toes every few seconds which might in turn produce back pain. The way to do it most efficiently would be to stop erector spinae working and, therefore, to lie on the floor supine and raise one's chest and pelvis at the same time by contracting the abdominal muscles which body builders and athletes do. Then a wonderful rippling anterior abdominal wall is produced, unattainable in the ordinary mortal (Fig. 2.11). All these spinal muscles are fired by peripheral nerves branching from the *spinal cord*, as are, of course, the muscles of the arms and legs.

During foetal life the spinal cord runs down the whole spine to the bottom of the tail bone (*coccyx*). Then because of a greater growth rate in the bony spine, the bottom of the spinal cord gradually migrates upwards until at birth the bottom tip of the spinal cord (*the conus*) lies at the level of the intervertebral disc between the first and second lumbar vertebrae (the L1/2 level) (Figs 2.12a and 2.12b). Below this level, that is between L1/2 and the bottom of the coccyx, there are the terminal branches of the spinal cord. As they come off they travel vertically downwards and they look like a horse's tail and are, therefore, called the *cauda equina*.

At every intervertebral level, on each side, a branch comes out from the spinal cord to supply sensation and muscle power to its target area. As these branches leave the spinal cord they are called *nerve roots*. Thus, while each thoracic nerve root leaves the spine horizontally the lumbar and sacral roots have to travel obliquely or frankly longitudinally downwards from the bottom of the spinal cord before they exit. Therefore, the first sacral (S1) nerve root, which is commonly affected by a prolapsed intervertebral disc at the relevant level (the L5/S1 level),

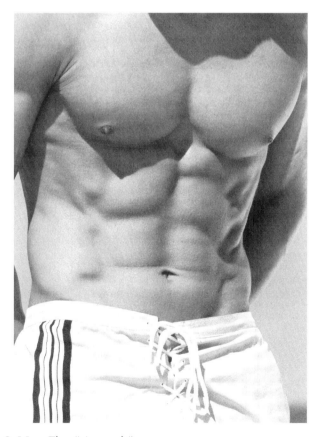

Fig. 2.11   The "six-pack".

has had to travel all the way down from about the waist before it finally makes its exit. This is important in the unfortunate individual with a serious spinal fracture–dislocation. In the thoracic region, the spinal cord fills most of the spinal canal,

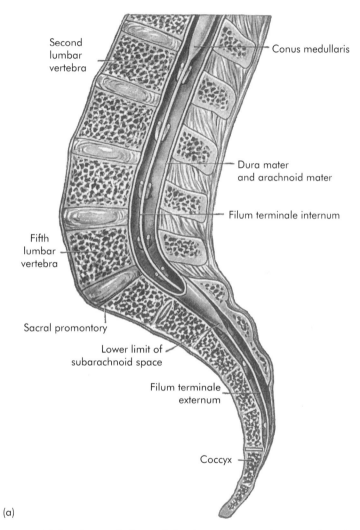

Second lumbar vertebra

Conus medullaris

Dura mater and arachnoid mater

Filum terminale internum

Fifth lumbar vertebra

Sacral promontory

Lower limit of subarachnoid space

Filum terminale externum

Coccyx

(a)

Fig. 2.12(a) Sagittal slice of the lower spine showing that the end of the spinal cord (the conus) lies at the junction of the first and second lumbar vertebrae. The fibrous filum then carries on to the coccyx (the nerves of the cauda equina have been removed for clarity). From Gray's Anatomy (1989). Eds Williams PL, Warwick R, Dyson M, Bannister LM. Thirty-Seventh Edition. Churchill Livingstone. Edinburgh & London.

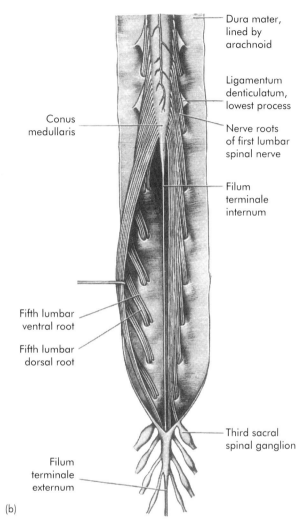

Dura mater,
lined by
arachnoid

Ligamentum
denticulatum,
lowest process

Conus
medullaris

Nerve roots
of first lumbar
spinal nerve

Filum
terminale
internum

Fifth lumbar
ventral root

Fifth lumbar
dorsal root

Third sacral
spinal ganglion

Filum
terminale
externum

(b)

Fig. 2.12(b) Front view of lower spine showing how the lower spinal cord gives rise to all the nerve roots that carry on therefrom referred to as the cauda equina. From Gray's Anatomy (1989). Eds Williams PL, Warwick R, Dyson M, Bannister LM. Thirty-Seventh Edition. Churchill Livingstone. Edinburgh & London.

whereas below the conus, where the cauda equina is, the nerve roots only occupy a fraction of the cross-sectional area. Therefore, if a spinal dislocation occurs at the eleventh thoracic level, for example, then there is a real risk of complete paralysis of the function of all the nerves below that level which would include complete loss of sensation, motor power, bladder and

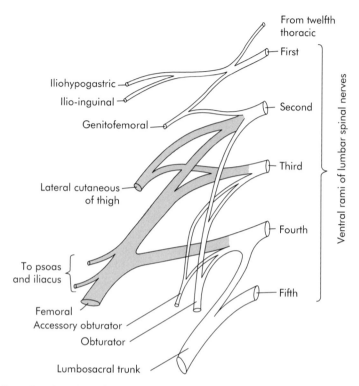

Fig. 2.13 *Spaghetti junction.* The lumbar nerves divide, rejoin and divide again to form the lumbar plexus. From Gray's Anatomy (1989). Eds Williams PL, Warwick R, Dyson M, Bannister LM. Thirty-Seventh Edition. Churchill Livingstone. Edinburgh & London.

bowel function. If, however, the dislocation occurred at the L3 level then even with major displacement many nerve roots may be spared with a more benign prognosis and this we refer to as *lumbar root escape.* Moreover, the nerve roots are much more resilient than the spinal cord.

In the thoracic region, after the spinal nerve roots pass horizontally out of the spinal canal, they supply a band of tissue rather like a stripe around the chest. However, in the cervical and lumbar regions outside the spine the nerve roots are repeatedly joined together and branch rather like *spaghetti junction* before going on to supply the muscles and the skin of the limbs (Fig. 2.13). Not surprisingly, the spinal cord is enlarged in the cervical and lumbar regions where these branches come off and have to travel long distances. As each nerve root does supply a certain part with feeling and with muscle power, surgeons in turn can, by examining the arms and legs, for instance, know from which part of the spine the problem is originating. Once a nerve comes out of the spine, it is called a *mixed peripheral nerve* because it contains nerve fibres of different sorts – those that might supply sensation (*sensory nerves*), those that do odd things entirely autonomously without conscious control like make blood vessels contract and dilate, or make your hair stand on end, or make you sweat (*autonomic nerves*) and those that supply power to muscles (*motor nerves*).

Suffice it to say at this stage that many years ago neurophysiologists mapped out on the arms and legs the distribution of individual nerve roots. Medical students do learn them, general practitioners (GPs) might know them, registrars in training should know them and consultant spinal surgeons must know them (Fig. 2.14). These maps look rather like maps of countries divided into counties and thus, if you know that Sussex is supplied by the fifth lumbar nerve root (L5) and the patient complains of reduced sensation in the Sussex region then you can begin to incriminate pressure on the L5 nerve root. These sensory distributions of individual nerve roots are called *dermatomes*. Meanwhile, if the first sacral nerve root (S1) supplies Surrey and the patient has a sensation of painful pins and needles in the Surrey area then that would alert suspicion to the S1 nerve root. Each nerve root also tends to supply particular muscle groups, *myotomes*, and if the area of reduced sensation in Sussex was accompanied by weakness of the ability to *extend* (lift up) the toes then this would also incriminate the L5 nerve root as it preferentially supplies motor power to the muscles which extend the toes and foot. If, therefore, we have someone with a disc prolapse pressing on the L5 nerve root then a *drop foot* can be a serious consequence.

- Dermatome – area of skin supplied by a particular nerve root
- Myotome – muscle groups supplied by a particular nerve root

The brain and spinal cord are surrounded by three sleeves (*maters*) of fibrous tissue (Fig. 2.15), the inner two being very flimsy but the outer sleeve, called the dura, is substantial and has

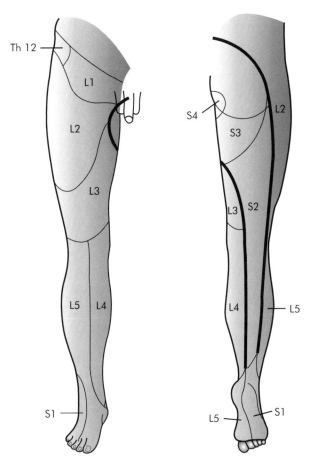

Fig. 2.14 *The dermatome maps of the lower extremities.* These are the sensory distributions on the skin of the various nerves that go to the legs. For instance, L1 supplies the front of the thigh just below the groin whereas both L5 and S1 get as far as the foot. Disc surgery is principally concerned with the L4, 5 and S1 roots.

a very important biomechanical function. It also surrounds the cauda equina, and as each nerve root emerges from the spine the dura gives it a tubular covering for a short distance, as the beginning of the arms would be by a short-sleeved sports shirt. Between the brain, spinal cord, nerve roots and the dural sheath is the cerebro-spinal fluid, which has a number of important functions, one of which is the mechanical protection of the nerve tissue it surrounds. In this regard, it resembles how the air in an inflated car tyre protects the rim of the wheel. If, however,

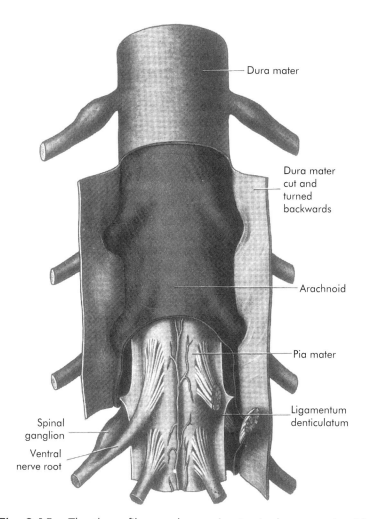

Fig. 2.15   The three fibrous sleeves (maters), dura, arachnoid and pia, which surround the spinal cord and cauda equina. From Gray's Anatomy (1989). Eds Williams PL, Warwick R, Dyson M, Bannister LH. Thirty-Seventh Edition. Churchill Livingstone. Edinburgh & London.

the tyre has a puncture the rim is no longer protected; if there is a dural tear then the local nerve tissue is immediately denied its buffering protective fluid surround as the cerebro-spinal fluid leaks out and the dura lies immediately against the underlying nerve tissue just as the deflated tyre wall would lie against the rim. Should this happen traumatically, for example at surgery, either deliberately when the dura is opened to take out an

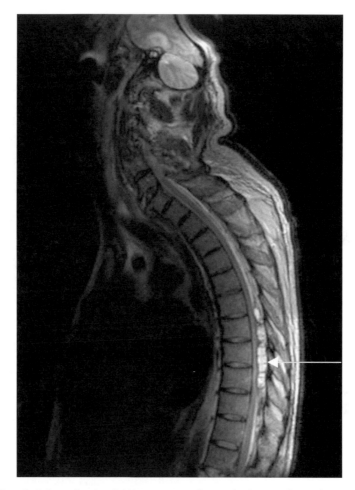

Fig. 2.16 Sagittal MRI section through the neck and upper thoracic spine showing blood (arrowed) in the canal compressing the cord. The patient was elderly and was on anticoagulant treatment for heart disease, thus favouring bleeding.

intradural tumour, or unexpectedly at, say, disc surgery, then this biomechanical danger must be appreciated. Wherever the surgeon goes, he leaves a trail of blood and if post-operative bleeding is substantial then a collection of blood can form which is called a *haematoma*. If this haematoma was formed from bleeding from the bone, ligaments or muscles around the spine and it lies outside the dura, it is called an *epidural* haematoma (Fig. 2.16). If the dura is intact and, therefore, resembles the fully inflated tyre, the nerve tissue is protected. Even with an intact dural tube, an expanding epidural haematoma does have the ability to cause nerve compression but it generally takes 6 or 7 days for that amount of pressure to overcome the fully inflated tyre situation. If, however, there is a dural leak then the time frame for significant nerve compression can be a matter of a few hours and generally not more than a day before manifesting itself clinically. Of course, the ideal situation is to get one's puncture repair outfit out and repair or patch the dural breach but that may not always be practicable with a large defect and a sound repair may not be a hundred per cent waterproof (cerebro-spinal fluid is like machine oil and will leak out given any opportunity). The consequences of post-operative nerve pressure are appreciable throughout the spine but are particularly well known in the lumbar region with the cauda equina. Sufficient epidural haematoma can build up compressing many of the nerve roots of the cauda equina including those supplying bladder and bowel. Adequate neurological monitoring of the post-operative spine patient is, therefore, mandatory.

Perhaps this is not a bad time to introduce some of the requirements in "Good Medical Practice" by the General Medical Council (GMC). In its remit to "protect patients and guide doctors", the GMC has produced this pamphlet and updates it every few years. Every doctor registered by the GMC receives a copy of this pamphlet and, reciprocally, you cannot practise without being registered with the GMC and, therefore, as a doctor you cannot avoid receiving this document. It does not just concern "Aims" and "Suggestions" but "Duties" and "Musts". The following are the relevant entries in "Good Medical Practice" that pertain to monitoring patients clinically. These are selected extracts but readers, who are not medically registered can easily obtain a copy from the GMC as the pamphlet "Good Medical Practice" is firmly in the public domain.

"Good Clinical Care"

Good clinical care must include

- an adequate assessment of the patient's condition, based on the history and clinical signs and, if necessary, an appropriate examination.

In providing care you must

- keep clear, accurate and contemporaneous patient records which report the relevant clinical findings, the decisions made and the information given to patients;
- keep colleagues well informed when sharing the care of patients.

Arranging cover

You must be satisfied that, when you are off duty, suitable arrangements are made for your patient's medical care. These arrangements should include effective hand-over procedures and clear communication between doctors.

Delegation and referral

Delegation involves asking a nurse, doctor, medical student or other health care worker to provide treatment or care on your behalf. When you delegate care or treatment you must be sure that the person to whom you delegate is competent to carry out the procedure or provide the therapy involved. You must always pass on enough information about the treatment needed. You will still be responsible for the overall management of the patient.

When you refer a patient, you should provide all relevant information about the patient's history and current condition.

Good Medical Practice is quite explicit

- You must make an adequate assessment of your patient's condition.
- You must keep clear accurate and contemporaneous records.
- You must keep colleagues well informed when sharing the care of patients.
- You must be satisfied that when you are off duty suitable arrangements are made for your patient's medical care.

Delegation involves asking someone else to provide treatment on your behalf. You must always pass on enough

(continued)

> information about the patient and the treatment needed. You will still be responsible for the overall management of the patient.
>
> When you refer a patient you should provide all relevant information about the patient's history and current condition.
>
> Not to do so is by definition not **Good Clinical Practice**.

As we have seen, the bony spine is a long, gently curved mechanical structure which is a glorified cylinder containing the spinal cord and its branches. Although it is divided up into 33 blocks of bone (*vertebrae*), developmental fusion of the sacral and coccygeal segments means that we are left with seven cervical vertebrae, twelve thoracic, five lumbar, one sacral and one (usually) coccygeal (Fig. 2.10). Apart from the first cervical joint, and the sacro-coccygeal joint, the remaining vertebrae are separated by intervertebral discs.

Each vertebra has a basically similar shape in cross section. If we start off with a lumbar vertebra this has a *body* in front which is fairly chunky, wide from side to side, slightly kidney shaped, and would do, with a bit of latitude, for a house (Fig. 2.9a). The house has a sloping roof made up of the *laminae* on each side. They meet at the top in the mid-line where there is a bony projection called the *spinous process*. The roof of the house is attached to the house by a *pedicle* on each side. Where the pedicle and laminae join there is a bony projection sideways called the *transverse* process. The house itself has strong but slender walls of cortical bone and the house itself contains some honeycomb trabecular bone and red marrow. We said that the spine was a glorified cylinder containing nerve tissue and the nerve tissue is in the attic, under the roof, and not in the house. Each nerve root passes out between adjacent roofs, between adjacent pedicles to be precise (Fig. 2.9b).

The symphysis (joint) between adjacent vertebral bodies contains the intervertebral disc which degenerates throughout life, in varying degrees in varying individuals mostly due to genetic programming, and as a result the nucleus in the disc

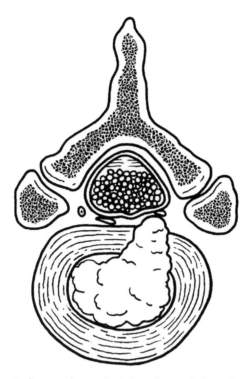

Fig. 2.17 A disc prolapse bulging through into the attic. From Operative Spinal Surgery (1991). Eds Torrens MJ, Dickson RA. Churchill Livingstone. Edinburgh & London.

can bulge (protrude) or even prolapse through the surrounding fibrous annulus. This latter is a *disc hernia*. It can herniate in any direction. It can go anteriorly (down into the cellar), sideways (into the garden path) or posteriorly (upwards into the attic). As it is the attic that contains the clockwork (the nerves), posterior disc prolapses can produce neurological problems (Fig. 2.17).

The vertebral bodies are more heart shaped in cross section in the thoracic spine, as opposed to more squat cervical and lumbar vertebral body cross sections, and there are minor variations in other anatomical parameters but the essence of the construct is that the spine is like a crane (Fig. 2.18) with the jib of the crane being the vertebral bodies in front, while the cables of the crane are the muscles and ligaments attached to the spinous and transverse processes on the roof of the house (Figs 2.9 and 2.19). It can be clearly seen from such a construct that

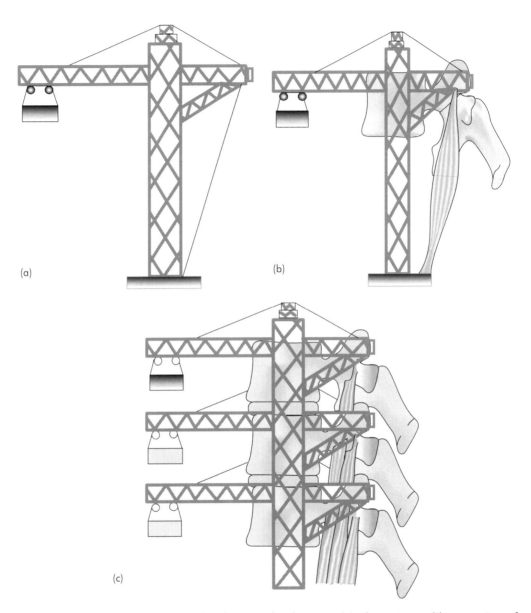

Fig. 2.18 (a) A typical crane. (b) The vertebral crane. (c) The spine is like a series of cranes. From Harms J, Tabasso G (1999). Instrumented Spinal Surgery. Principles and Technique. Thieme, Stuttgart & New York.

these are terraced houses with adjacent houses, separated by discs, which would tend to resist *compressive forces* (squeezing) like the jib of the crane, while the ligaments and muscles attached to the flagpoles sticking out of the roof would be the

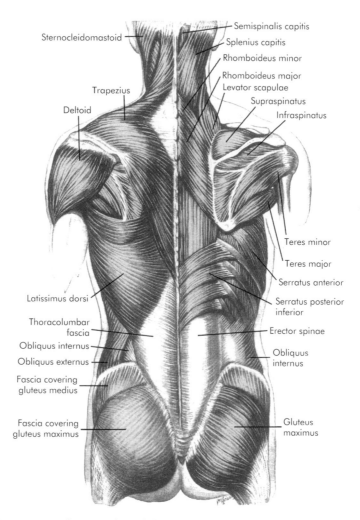

Fig. 2.19 The muscles of the back are lashed onto the spinous and transverse processes. From Gray's Anatomy (1989). Eds Williams PL, Warwick R, Dyson M, Bannister LH. Thirty-Seventh Edition. Churchill Livingstone. Edinburgh & London.

tension members, like the cables of the crane, and resist *tension* or stretching. We shall go into the relevant biomechanics in more detail in the strain and injury sections but it can be seen that the spine is very well suited for its important functions of providing a strong supportive framework, protecting important organs and in particular the spinal cord, as well as its metabolic and haematological functions (in the young the vertebral body marrow produces blood cells). Moreover, it is provided with multiple links so that it can carry out these functions just as optimally in a very wide range of positions.

SUGGESTIONS FOR FURTHER READING

Grant's Method of Anatomy. A Clinical Problem-Solving Approach, Eleventh edition. Basmajian JV, Slonecker CE. Williams & Wilkins International Edition, 1989.

Last's Anatomy: Regional and Applied, Tenth edition. Sinnatamby, Chummy S. Churchill Livingstone, 1999.

Clinically Oriented Anatomy, Fourth edition. Keith, PhD, Moore, Arthur F. Dalley II. Paperback 1164 pages (April 1999) Lippincott, Williams & Wilkins.

Three great anatomy teaching texts, a fraction of the size of Gray or Cunningham; a knowledge of either would get you through the Fellow of the Royal College of Surgeons (FRCS) anatomy examinations! Therefore, far too detailed for the lay person but well worth having in your library to dip into from time to time.

Clinical Anatomy: A Revision and Applied Anatomy for Clinical Students, Ninth edition. Ellis H. Blackwell Scientific, Oxford, 1997.

A nice little text, not enough to get through the FRCS examination but a much easier read. Nonetheless, a bit too much for the non-medic.

Most personal injury work is musculo-skeletal and there really is not a suitable source of reference for, say, the busy lawyer, hence the reasonably comprehensive anatomical coverage in this (our) book, which we hope you are enjoying.

Biomechanics of the Spine

To support the body and provide a wide range of motion while protecting the spinal cord demands stable movements and the prevention of instability and the spine is brilliantly designed for these purposes. It is a column comprising a series of bone segments (vertebrae) separated by discs and joined by ligaments so that considerable movement of the whole is produced by relatively small displacements at many sites rather like a bicycle chain. This is a much more *stable* configuration than motion occurring at few very mobile joints as in the limbs. Notwithstanding, the spine can be damaged.

The ability of a structure to resist breakage depends upon two things – its shape (*geometry*) and what it is made of (*materials*) and bones including vertebrae are no exceptions.

Most matters that concern doctors and lawyers in personal injury or medical negligence are to do with the effects of trauma, which is what happens to the body in response to an applied load, and, therefore, it is necessary to become familiar with some of the more important biomechanical words and phrases. We have already seen that when something is squashed, it is under *compression*; and when something is stretched, it is under *tension*. Compression and tension are, therefore, forces applied along the length of the material. The third type of force, *shear*, is applied to the side of the material at right angles to the long axis, rather like rubbing something.

- Compression – squeezing
- Tension – stretching
- Shear – rubbing

Then *stress* and *strain* are commonly used words and stress means pressure, while strain is the amount that a material that is compressed or stretched is deformed by a given stress.

Therefore, the *stiffness* of a material describes how it strains in proportion to the stress applied to it. Stiffer materials move less for a given load. When the spine is compressed the discs bulge (a bit) because they are less stiff than the bone on each side, indeed approximately one hundred times so. That is why *normal* discs bulge beyond the confines of the vertebrae on each side and so a disc bulge is the normal state of affairs. As we shall see, when discs degenerate they become much stiffer. You can squeeze normal discs a bit but the proposition that the more degenerate a disc becomes the more you can squeeze the nucleus out is not only quite unfounded but is exactly the opposite of what actually happens.

Stiffness, of course, should not be confused with *strength*, which is the amount of load the material can take before *failure* (when it breaks) and when the spine continues to be compressed to breaking point (something has to give) it is always bone that fractures before the disc would break (Fig. 3.1). This is because bone is very much weaker than disc. Moreover, because these are *essential physical principles*, it is not possible for discs to break before bone (disc is stronger) in the same way that it is not possible for bone to bulge more than disc (bone is stiffer). Precisely,

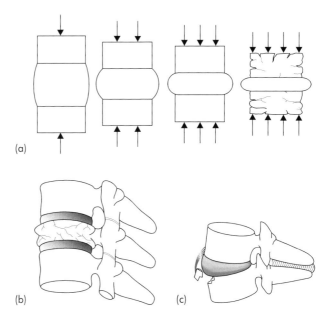

Fig. 3.1   (a) When the spine is compressed to failure the intervening disc bulges a bit because it is less stiff than the bone on each side but when the stresses carry on rising bone breaks first because it is weaker than disc. The disc does not squash down anywhere near as much as depicted in real life. (b) That is why compression fractures occur because bone is weaker than disc. (c) Similarly, ligament is stronger than bone and when the spine is extended to failure a piece of bone is pulled off by the stronger ligament. From Radin EL, Blaha SD, Rose RM, Litsky AS (1992). Practical Biomechanics for the Orthopaedic Surgeon. Second Edition. Churchill Livingstone. Edinburgh & London.

the same principles apply when the spinal column is stretched. Discs narrow and stretch in tension (a bit) just as they shorten and bulge (a bit) in compression. The amount of stiffness is just the same in tension as in compression and again bone stretches much less than disc does because it is stiffer. Discs also have the ability to continue to strain with time albeit very gradually. Living on this planet under the influence of gravity we become more than a centimetre shorter during the day and regain our height in the morning after a good night's sleep. This time-dependent change in shape is called *creep*. This change in disc height takes hours and reciprocally no significant change in disc height occurs in response to discreet loads, for example, jumping up and down on the spot.

Similarly, bone is weaker than ligament in tension just as it is in compression. When the spinal column is stretched to breaking point, the ligaments that hold the spine together pull off a piece of bone to which they are attached. The outer annulus is effectively the ligament of the disc. Bone is weaker than ligament in all circumstances and, therefore, bone fails first. Again these are strict physical principles and because ligaments are vastly stronger in tension than bone then not only does bone break first but the possibility of ligaments breaking first is simply not an option.

If the spinal column does break, say with the extreme violence of a high-speed road-traffic accident, and if all the supporting structures are disrupted, displacement may occur (subluxation or frank dislocation) (Figs 2.7 and 6.6). The area of disruption is not as stiff as an intact spine and so more deformation can occur in the area of injury.

Consequently, *unstable* spinal injuries must not be allowed to displace and should be stabilised as soon as possible lest local deformation disrupts the spinal cord. Reciprocally, and for the same reason of lesser stiffness, displaced injuries can be reduced and realigned by traction or the insertion of metalwork (Figs 3.2a and 3.2b).

Horizontal (shear) forces are also resisted by the ligaments of the spine, their individual fibres being obliquely plaited together, again making bone much weaker than ligament in response to shear. The *posterior facet joints* can also help to resist shear forces. These are the joints linking the bottom of the roofs of successive terraced houses and in the lumbar region they are orientated

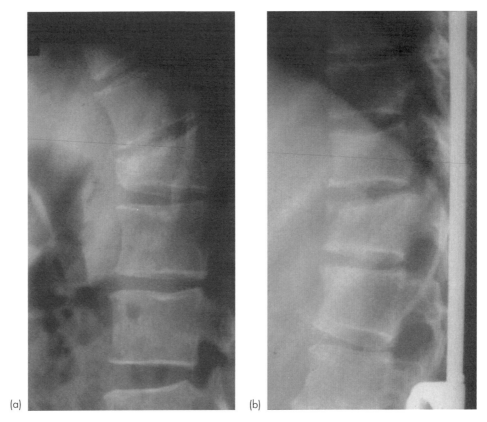

(a)   (b)

Fig. 3.2 A thoraco-lumbar fracture–dislocation reduced by the application of metalwork. (a) After reduction pre-operative lateral X-ray showing the deformed vertebra. (b) By the application of metalwork, height has been considerably restored.

vertically (Fig. 3.3). If you look at the spine from the back they look like book-ends (with no books in between), although there is a very small joint space. It is clear that any twisting of the back is promptly met by the book-ends coming together and, thus, the lumbar spine is well protected in this regard as of course are the lumbar discs.

Due to its anatomy and physiology the spinal column bends, and like any other column, material on the convex side is under tension and that on the concave side is under compression with a line down the middle where there are no stresses (the *neutral axis*) (Fig. 3.4). That is why long bones can be hollow, because the neutral axis is where you biomechanically require least material. When we pick up a weight, our spine is not simply compressed or stretched but also bends and the outer surfaces

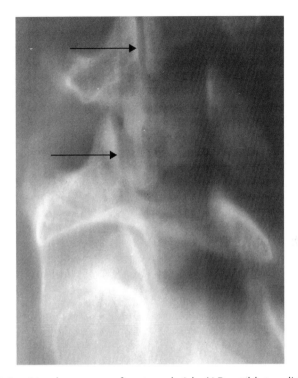

Fig. 3.3 You have seen front and side (AP and lateral) X-rays of the spine but this is an oblique view (half-way between AP and lateral) which is useful for looking at the facet joints (arrowed) and the bone in between them. Compare with Fig. 5.2.

are where the biggest stresses occur and these are referred to as the *extreme fibres*.

Thus, a common fracture pattern in the neck is a hyperextension injury. The avulsion of a small piece of bone from the top or bottom of the adjacent vertebra confirms that under maximum tension bone is weaker than ligament (Fig. 3.1). For the same reasons as already articulated, the other possibility (ligament breaking first) is simply not on the cards.

There are many different spinal ligaments; for example, the ligaments joining the tops of the houses (supraspinous ligaments) and the elastic ligaments joining the laminae (ligamenta flava) (Fig. 2.8). Not only are the different posterior ligamentous structures at different distances from the neutral axis but they also have different stiffnesses and are able to *load-share*. Thus, the ligament furthest from the neutral axis does not do all the

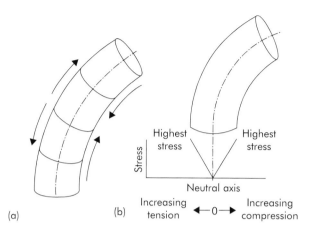

Fig. 3.4   When a column is bent, then the material on the concave side is under compression and on the concave side under tension. The middle of the column, the neutral axis is not subjected to any force while material on the convex and concave edges, the extreme fibres, are under maximum stress. From Radin EL, Blaha SD, Rose RM, Litsky AS (1992). Practical Biomechanics for the Orthopaedic Surgeon. Second Edition. Churchill Livingstone. New York & Edinburgh.

work. Think about what happens when the posterior elements are removed as a necessary part of a *laminectomy* (unroofing the spine from the back) operation and are consequently replaced by scar tissue whose stiffness characteristics are quite inappropriate, and when the posterior muscles are weakened or denervated by surgery (Fig. 3.5). Stress concentrations can then rise, because scar cannot load-share like the original anatomy.

In addition, the abdominal cavity acts like a water-filled balloon and its hydrostatic pressure supports the loads on the spine (Fig. 3.6). Consequently, obesity, multiple abdominal operations or pregnancies produce abdominal muscle laxity and make the abdominal cavity much less biomechanically effective. Therefore, what a corset is supposed to be doing is obvious although it clearly has to be so tight as to be very uncomfortable before it can work properly in this manner (incontinence may then be an unfortunate side-effect!).

Discs act as intervertebral spacers, separating adjacent vertebrae, thus, facilitating the great range of motion that the spine enjoys. In so doing the bending forces on the bony parts of the spine are minimised and the spine can, thus, bend at much lower stresses. If a disc degenerates (natural process of genetic

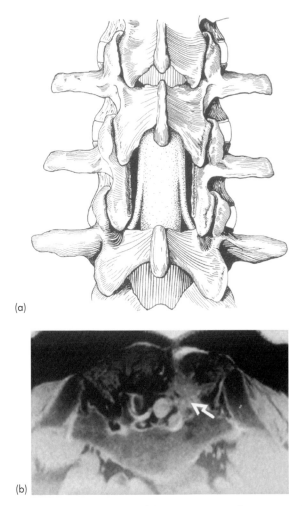

(a)

(b)

Fig. 3.5 (a) The amount of bone removed in an ordinary laminectomy and, therefore, the amount of space that will be filled in by post-operative scar tissue with quite different physical properties from that which it replaced. From Operative Spinal Surgery (1991). Eds Torrens MS, Dickson RA. Churchill Livingstone. Edinburgh & London. (b) Axial post-laminectomy MRI images showing a mass of scar tissue replacing everything that was removed or traumatised (arrow).

self-destruction), however, then motion is lost and stress concentration occurs at adjacent joints. This is the same principle as fusion, internal fixation or *spondylosis* (natural wear and tear arthritis) increasing local stiffness and producing increased stress in nearby joints (Fig. 3.7). This is very much more theoretical than practical and, while a long fusion for a spinal

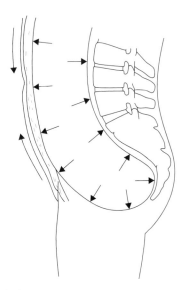

Fig. 3.6 The abdominal balloon helps to support the spine. From Radin EL, Blaha SD, Rose RM, Litsky AS (1992). Practical Biomechanics for the Orthopaedic Surgeon. Second Edition. Churchill Livingstone. New York & Edinburgh.

deformity in a child may well cause painful arthritis at adjacent joints in later life, the proposition that a one-level lumbar fusion will affect nearby joints in any meaningfully clinical way is quite unfounded.

One of the primary mechanisms of stress relief in the skeleton is the insertion of joints in the right places rather like articulations in the roadway of a bridge. When you drive over, for example, the Forth road bridge you will feel that you go over, every so often, a gap or joint in the road surface. This is to allow movement and stress to escape (Fig. 3.8). In addition, muscles that straddle joints act as guy wires and reduce bending stresses by increasing the compressive stresses in bone (Fig. 3.9). Bone is like concrete – it is good in compression but not in tension and, therefore, it can take an increase in compressive stress as a good trade-off.

In injuries it is not just the weight of the object or person that matters but its speed as well. It is really the *energy* considerations that matter. Energy is the ability of an object to do work, while work is the expenditure of energy. *Kinetic energy* is energy produced by motion (the faster you go the greater the energy)

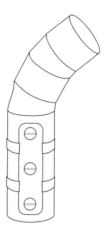

Fig. 3.7 A plate with three screws has been applied to fuse the bottom two joints of the spine. Increased stresses will, therefore, be taken on the articulation above but the notion that this will inevitably lead to clinically significant and accelerated degenerative change is quite unproven particularly as most fusions in elective practice are carried out for degenerative conditions which pathology often affects adjacent levels. So-called "acceleration" at an adjacent level is more than likely the natural history of the underlying condition. A fusion three times as long might have some effect but the evidence that a one- or two-level fusion does this is unconvincing. From Radin EL, Blaha SD, Rose RM, Litsky AS (1992). Practical Biomechanics for the Orthopaedic Surgeon. Second Edition. Churchill Livingstone. New York & Edinburgh.

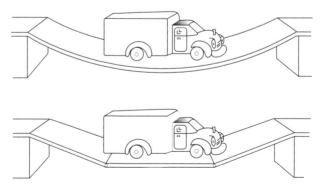

Fig. 3.8 The insertion of joints in a bridge allows movement and stresses to escape, thus, protecting the integrity of the overall construct. From Radin EL, Blaha SD, Rose RM, Litsky AS (1992). Practical Biomechanics for the Orthopaedic Surgeon. Second Edition. Churchill Livingstone. New York & Edinburgh.

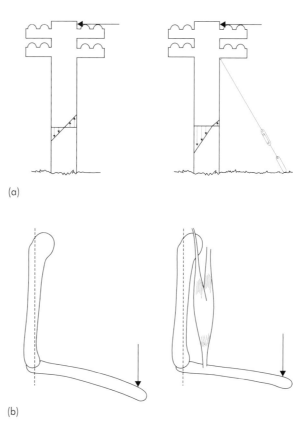

(a)

(b)

Fig. 3.9   (a) If a high-tension cable pylon (or even a telegraph pole) is subject to a strong prevailing wind in the direction of the arrow then the addition of a simple cable will reduce bending and increase compressive forces, which the pylon is much better able to resist than tension (back to tent poles/guy ropes and masts/rigging!). (b) Similarly, an important function of muscles is not just to contract to flex a joint, but also to resist elongation, thus, protecting a joint as the biceps does in this example protecting the elbow. From Radin EL, Blaha SD, Rose RM, Litsky AS (1992). Practical Biomechanics for the Orthopaedic Surgeon. Second Edition. Churchill Livingstone. New York & Edinburgh.

while *potential* energy is energy produced by height (the higher you fall the more energy applied when you hit the ground).

- Energy – the ability to do work
- Work – the expenditure of energy
- Kinetic energy – energy produced by movement
- Potential energy – energy produced by height

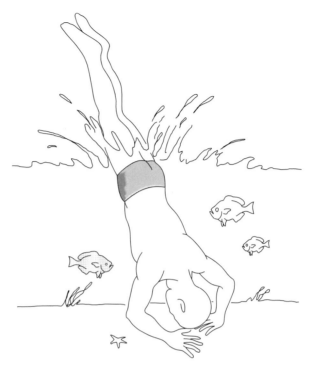

Fig. 3.10 Unfortunately, shallow water does not decelerate you enough to dissipate the energy of the dive. Deep end best. From Radin EL, Blaha SD, Rose RM, Litsky AS (1992). Practical Biomechanics for the Orthopaedic Surgeon. Second Edition. Churchill Livingstone. New York & Edinburgh.

Newton told us that for every action there is an equal and opposite reaction and it is this reaction force when an object may be rapidly decelerated that dissipates energy and can produce injury. If you dive into a swimming pool at the shallow end there is not enough water to decelerate you and you can break your neck (Fig. 3.10), unlike what happens in the deep end, when you decelerate through a substantial depth of water, although of course you can drown in the process!

A boxer, who may know nothing about biomechanics, learns or is trained to *ride a punch*. He sees the punch coming and if he cannot get out of the way of it, sways backwards so as to allow the energy of the punch to be dissipated over distance and, thus, time. By contrast, the boxer who does not see the punch coming may be unable to move or indeed may be moving forwards into the punch in which case there is little or no time to dissipate the energy with a resultant knock-out. Wicket

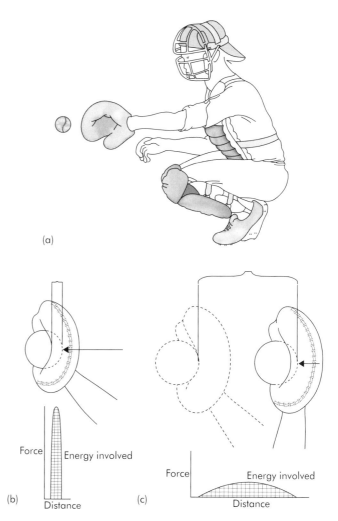

Fig. 3.11   (a) The catcher at baseball wears a glove of considerable thickness so that the applied force is attenuated over some distance. (b) If the catching hand remains stationary, the energy can still be very high. (c) Accordingly, the catcher moves his arm backwards as the ball is caught. Out-field cricketers do the same, when they catch the ball and then bring it towards their chest. From Radin EL, Blaha SD, Rose RM, Litsky AS (1992). Practical Biomechanics for the Orthopaedic Surgeon. Second Edition. Churchill Livingstone. New York & Edinburgh.

keepers wear padded gloves so that energy can be absorbed before it reaches the hand and the same sort of rationale is behind wearing padding, if you are a rugby player or American football player and why baseball players have that seemingly ridiculously big glove on their catching hand (Fig. 3.11). It is

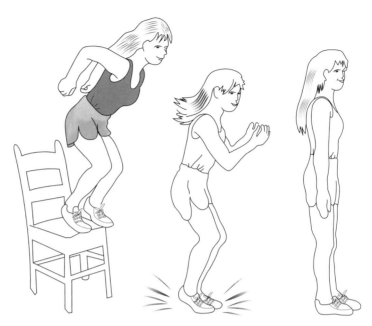

Fig. 3.12 When we jump down with our hips, knees and ankles flexed, we then extend these joints to dissipate the applied energy. From Radin EL, Blaha SD, Rose RM, Litsky AS (1992). Practical Biomechanics for the Orthopaedic Surgeon. Second Edition. Churchill Livingstone. New York & Edinburgh.

this dissipation of energy or *shock absorption* that is crucial in preventing skeletal and spinal injury.

As regards the spine, the muscles and ligaments play a very important role in absorbing the energy of an impact because the stresses cause movement and as the spine can accept considerable deformations, the stretching of the muscles and ligaments is optimised to take the strain. So the tensile forces in the muscles, ligaments and tendons can be transformed into compressive forces across the vertebral bodies and discs, which they are far better able to accept than tensile loads, just as we saw with the telegraph pole (Fig. 3.9). And so we come to the same common denominator, namely, that shock absorption occurs by the peak shocks and loads created by sudden accelerations and decelerations being reduced to acceptable levels by increasing the distance over which the energy is dissipated. Most of us can jump from a height of about 6 ft onto a firm surface without causing injury and we do this by dissipating the energy by extending our hips, knees and ankles after impact (Fig. 3.12). The stiffer the landing, the shorter the time for energy dissipation and the higher the impact forces. Of course, *fatigue* means that the musculo-ligamentous systems above mentioned cannot react with the necessary speed and thus fitness for sports is a critical factor in resisting injury.

Most soft tissue injuries are caused not by muscles stretching beyond their limits but by stretching or even frank tearing, if they are subjected to forced stretching while they are actually contracting and this is typical of the hamstring tear or Achilles tendon rupture. Hence, the importance for, say, professional soccer players (or indeed any of us doing sports) to deliberately stretch their muscles, and warm up, before going on the field. Interestingly, it is not just stretching when cold that matters but also stretching again after activity when the muscles are warm with blood. Post-exercise stretching has a marked preventative effect on exercise-induced stiffness – try it and see!

SUGGESTIONS FOR FURTHER READING

Practical Biomechanics for the Orthopaedic Surgeon, Second edition. Radin E. Churchill Livingstone, 1992.

A god-send for the innumerate non-scientist by one of the great orthopaedic teachers in the world, Eric Radin. Although this is a primer it would probably get all orthopaedic trainees through their final fellowship of the Royal College of Surgeons in Orthopaedic Surgery. Wonderfully easy to read which is, of course, so notoriously difficult to write.

Structures – or Why Things Don't Fall Down. Gordon. Penguin Books, England, 1987.

Professor Gordon was Professor of Materials Technology at Reading University and wrote this fantastic book about materials, covering bridges, bent masonry columns in Salisbury Cathedral, bows, catapults and kangaroos, boilers, butts and Chinese junks, and the essential material science of the bias-cut nightie! Unputdownable. Try his other Penguin book – *The New Science of Strong Materials* – for just as good a bedtime read.

Degenerative Spinal Disease

With ageing, any part of the intervertebral joint can degener-ate and very often all parts do together. Thus, the intervertebral disc often degenerates in association with the posterior facet joints at the back. This is very much a genetically controlled process, and some individuals may have a relatively pristine spine at the age of 60, while others may have significant clini-cal features in childhood; such is the genetic hand we are all dealt at the moment of conception (Figs 4.1a and 4.1b).

Although intervertebral joints are symphyses and do not have an articular cartilage lining, the pathological changes going on in the disc with ageing are very similar to those occurring in the posterior facet joints behind, which are joints lined by hyaline

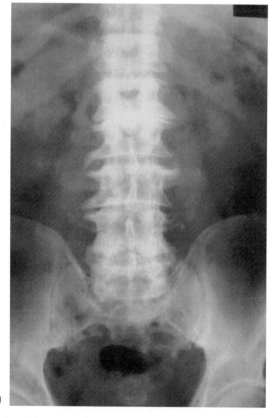

(a)

Fig. 4.1(a) AP X-ray showing widespread disc degeneration (disc space narrowing, bone thickening and spurs of new bone) throughout the lumbar spine.

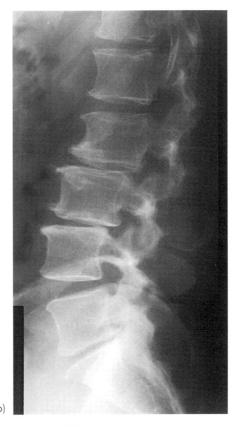

(b)

Fig. 4.1(b)   Lateral X-ray showing widespread disc degeneration (disc space narrowing, bone thickening and spurs of new bone) throughout the lumbar spine. Could be a 50- or 75-year old – depends on the hand you are dealt.

cartilage and degenerate in exactly the same way as other such cartilage-lined joints, for example the hip joint. There are two clinical effects from this process of degenerative spinal disease in the lumbar spine. The first is *spinal pain* and the second is *nerve root involvement*. If the process of nerve root involvement is just irritation, then there can be pain and tingling (pins and needles or *paraesthesiae*) along the course of the nerve. This often happens with a moderate-sized disc *hernia*. But if the nerve root involvement is frank compression of nerve substance, then there will be additional evidence of nerve dysfunction, such as loss of a reflex, reduction in power or loss of sensation. This commonly happens with a large disc hernia or if there is a piece of bone pressing on the nerve root.

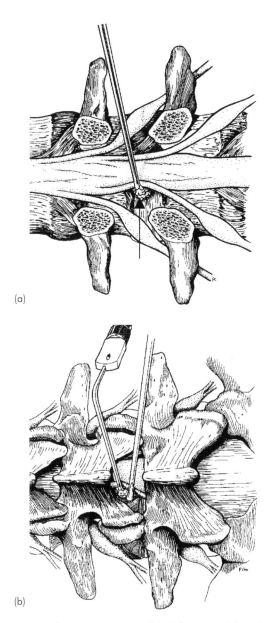

(a)

(b)

Fig. 4.2(a, b) *Nerve root decompression.* (a) After total laminectomy (for pictorial purposes only), the cauda equina and successive nerve roots can be seen with a disc hernia bulging a nerve root, which has been retracted towards the mid-line. (b) In practice, a total laminectomy is unnecessarily destructive. After a 1-in. skin incision centred radiographically over the relevant disc, the ligamentum flavum between adjacent laminae is excised, the nerve root located and retracted to expose the underlying disc hernia without much or any bone removal (preferably with the microscope). The spine is pictured sideways on – the way the surgeon sees it.

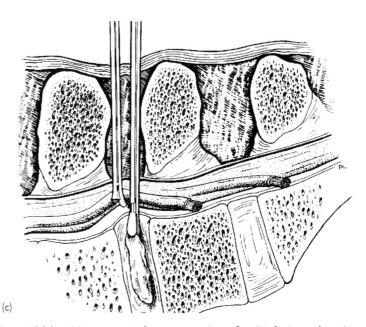

(c)

Fig. 4.2(c)   *Nerve root decompression*. Sagittal view showing that after the disc hernia has been excised only that tissue which is loose or can be easily mobilised using the discectomy forceps should be sacrificed. The disc space is not curetted in this operative procedure and a total discectomy is contraindicated. From Operative Spinal Surgery (1991). Eds Torrens MS, Dickson RA. Churchill Livingstone. Edinburgh & London.

Sometimes the tingling can be very uncomfortable and we call that *dysaesthesiae*. The site of spinal pain is much less precise an indicator of the origin of the problem than is the neurological expression; and so it is that if there is no nerve root involvement, then it can be very difficult to localise where the problem is coming from, particularly, if the radiological evidence of degenerative change is fairly widespread as is often the case (look at Fig. 4.1 and see which joint you would put your money on).

Consequently, in terms of therapy, operative treatment is much less effective for spinal pain than it is for neurological involvement. Thus, the operation of so-called *discectomy* is really a misnomer. Rather it should be called *nerve root decompression* (Figs 4.2a, b and c) because disc surgery is specifically addressed at the nerve root involvement component of the problem and not the spinal pain. Furthermore, the whole disc is not excised, just that, often smallish, portion compressing the nerve root.

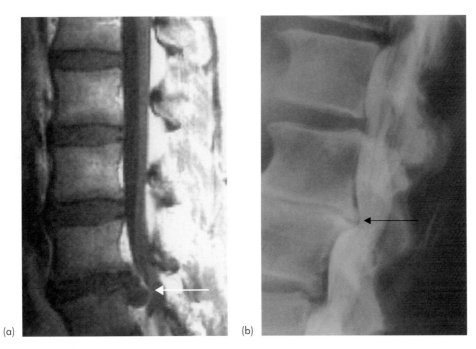

(a)   (b)

Fig. 4.3   (a) Sagittal MRI section showing a large disc hernia in a younger patient (arrow). (b) Sagittal myelogram (white dye injected into the cerebro-spinal fluid) showing spinal stenosis in an older patient with spurs of bone digging into the cauda equina (arrow).

It is useful to divide the time frame for the development of degenerative spinal disease into an early and a late phase, although, of course, it is a continuous process. The early phase of degeneration concerns the intervertebral disc and its concomitant change in shape (*herniation*) (Fig. 4.3a). Here the clinical expression tends to be less of spinal pain and more of nerve root involvement with often quite severe nerve root pain (*sciatica*) in the leg frequently of rapid onset; whereas in the older age group, degenerative spinal disease tends to be more insidious and neurological involvement more subtle with sciatica much less common. If the spine can be likened to a glorified cylinder, which conveys nerves, then the process of degenerative spinal disease with its concomitant new bone formation and disc bulging produces narrowing of the holes and canals through which nerves pass. This process is referred to as *spinal stenosis* (Fig. 4.3b). If it occurs in the main spinal canal (the attic), which conveys the spinal cord and cauda equina, then this tends to produce symptoms of *claudication* (cramps and tiredness in the legs which tend to be exercise related). This is called *central canal stenosis*. If it occurs more laterally, where the nerve roots pass out from the spine, then nerve root dysfunction may be the predominant factor. This is called *lateral recess* or *foraminal stenosis*.

Clearly biological age and genetic expression vary considerably, and so we do not uncommonly encounter a 40-year old with spinal stenosis and a 60-year old with a disc problem; and there is obviously some blurring as one phase moves into the other, but nonetheless the fundamental division into disc herniation or stenosis is a useful concept.

INTERVERTEBRAL DISC DEGENERATION

The phrase *slipped disc* is a rather unfortunate choice of words and would certainly suggest that first of all discs can slip out of place and perhaps secondly that they can be put back into place by, for instance, manipulative therapy. Nothing could be further from the truth. The term *disc herniation* is better, but is still misleading giving more of a physical sense to the process than the essentially natural and constitutional degenerative process that it really is. Intervertebral discs degenerate in much the same way that any other joint degenerates and, consequently, they share very much the same pathological process. This occurs to different degrees in different individuals, and as we shall see, as with primary osteoarthritis, is very much under genetic control with the physical environment having little or no part to play.

The process of degeneration is a biochemical one and has been well described. The nucleus inside the disc is gelatinous and contains clear viscous fluid. As degeneration proceeds, so this nucleus loses water and there is a relative increase in the amount of collagenous fibrous tissue. The dehydration process is well seen on magnetic resonance imaging (MRI) scans. A normal intervertebral disc contains a lot of water and, therefore, appears white like the cerebro-spinal fluid (Fig. 1.2a). There is a small central darker area in the nucleus, which looks like a hamburger in a bun. As degenerative dehydration proceeds and water is lost, the disc becomes darker and more

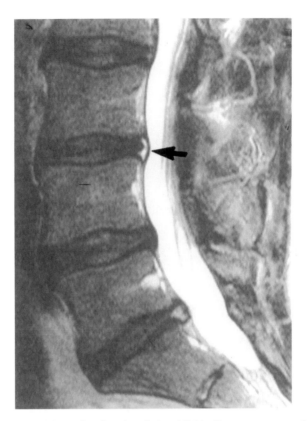

Fig. 4.4 HIZ at the back of the L3/4 disc seen as a bright area (arrow). Note the intact outer annulus of the disc behind it. This is often referred to as an annular tear, but clearly cannot be a result of trauma.

disorganised losing its hamburger-type appearance. This *disease* on the MRI scans seems to have some surgical appeal, but merely reflects the ongoing process of degeneration. The surrounding annulus also degenerates, and as it does so, clefts or fissures develop which can be seen on MRI scanning as high-intensity zones (HIZs). These are sometimes called *annular tears*; but again, like the phraseology slipped disc, erroneously implies a traumatic effect when these splits between adjacent annular fibres are part of the natural and constitutional degenerative process (Fig. 4.4). Indeed that there is an intact annular layer behind them confirms that they cannot be the result of a "tear". Milgram has wonderful pictures of the process of disc degeneration showing that the cellular changes must be constitutional (Fig. 4.5).

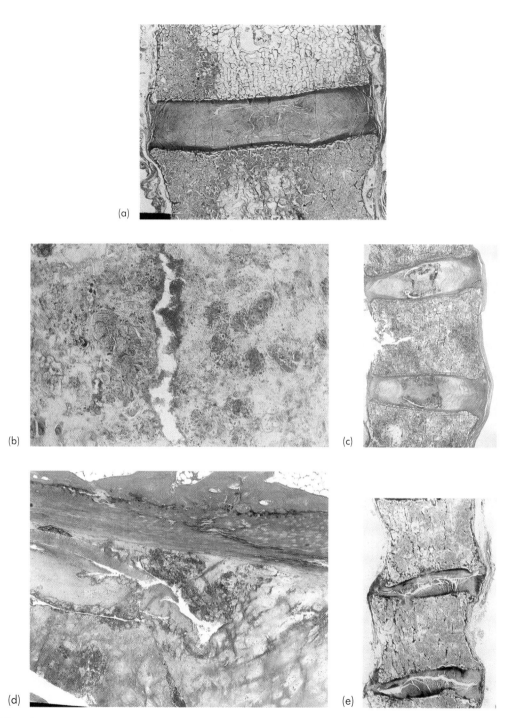

Fig. 4.5

Fig. 4.5 *(continued)*.

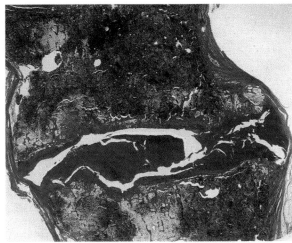

(f)

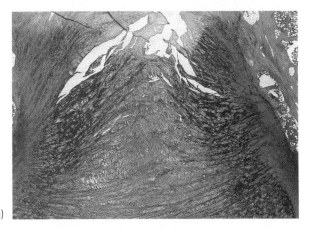

(g)

Fig. 4.5 Pathological sections from post-mortem specimens showing degenerative disc disease of varying severity. These magnificent illustrations are from Dr Milgram's wonderful pathology book (Radiologic and histologic pathology of non-tumorous, diseases of bones and joints), with kind permission from the publishers. (a) Mild degenerative disc disease in a 56-year-old man who died from cancer. The height of the disc is normal, but within its centre is a complex pattern of very small clefts (annular tears). (b) High-powered magnification of one of the clefts showing living cartilage cells within the region of disc degeneration. These cartilage cells may form nests similar to the cloning of cartilage cells in degenerated articular cartilage of synovial joints, such as the hip or knee. (c) Post-mortem spine of a 73-year-old male with no back pain. Two lumbar discs with adjacent vertebral bodies show central small clefts running parallel to the endplates. (d) Detail of one cleft showing purple degenerated matrix with some cartilage cell cloning. (e) Extensive cleft formation through both of the illustrated discs. (f) Detail of sequestrated disc showing gross clefts, which extend through the full sagittal width of the disc. (g) A peripheral annulus fibrosis tear. From Milgram JW (1990). Radiologic & Histologic Pathology of Non-tumorous Diseases of Bones and Joints. Northbrook Publishing.

As we have seen, intervertebral discs are less stiff than the bone on each side. Therefore, normal discs bulge a bit and, hence, disc bulging is a normal feature of scans. As the process of degeneration proceeds, however, disc bulging increases and does so in all directions because the height of the disc reduces with dehydration and the annulus, being more physically redundant, bulges. Down the middle of the back of the vertebral bodies and discs runs a strong ligament called the posterior longitudinal ligament (PLL) (Fig. 2.8); and this tends to deflect posterior disc bulging to one or other side (i.e. left or right), and this is the region of the nerve root (Fig. 4.6). Once big enough, and more focal than diffuse, this disc-bulging process is called *disc herniation*. You may have come across other words, such as *protrusion*, *prolapse* and *sequestration*, but they all refer to the same disc herniation process but reflect degree. A protrusion is less than a prolapse, and sequestration means that a bit of disc has actually become detached (sequestrated) and may lie free in the attic (Fig. 4.7).

- Intervertebral disc – spacer between adjacent vertebrae
  - Annulus fibrosus – tough outer layers
  - Nucleus pulposus – softer centre

(continued)

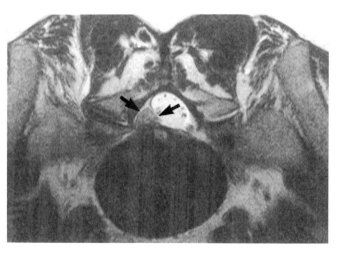

Fig. 4.6   Axial MRI showing a disc hernia (arrowed) deflected to one side by the PLL.

- Disc herniation – the nucleus bulges the annulus
  – Protrusion – bulging but not through the annulus
  – Prolapse – bulging through the annulus
  – Sequestration – loose piece of nucleus

We have already looked briefly at the clinical biomechanics of the spinal column, but now might be a good time to have a further look at this important subject, particularly, with reference to the intervertebral disc in relation to trauma. We have talked about tent poles, guy ropes, masts and rigging; and to get a composite picture of the biomechanics of the spinal column, it may be helpful to consider the spine as a crane (Fig. 2.18). The vertebral bodies at the front, which resist compressive loads, are the jib of the crane; while the muscles and ligaments at the back of the spine, which resist tension, are the cables of the crane. Meanwhile, the intervertebral disc is there to separate

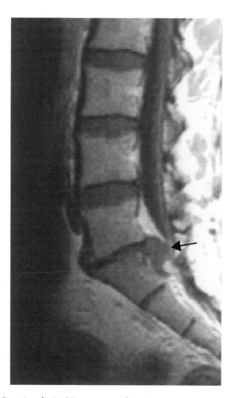

Fig. 4.7 Sagittal MRI scan showing a sequestrated disc fragment lying behind the body of S1 (arrow).

the jib into sections providing movement, which in turn allows the spine to perform its function over a considerable range. This in turn facilitates shock absorption, particularly, by the muscles and ligaments, which stretch to take the strain. An important function of the spinal column (perhaps the most important) is to protect the spinal cord and its branches during this considerable range of motion and in an environment, which is often extremely hostile. It simply would not do for discs to be popping out of place all the time, which would quickly make it almost impossible to encounter a normal disc on an MRI scan. There has been much biomechanical investigation carried out on the human spine as all orthopaedic surgeons, particularly those who claim any expertise in the spine, should know about. For instance, in the laboratory using cadaver lumbar spine joints which have been freshly excised from bodies and loaded in standard engineering testing machines, compression loading of such a spine to failure *always* produces vertebral body fractures irrespective of the rate of loading and the amount of applied load, and never produces disc failure (disc is stronger than bone) (Fig. 3.1).

Should the lumbar spine be twisted, then the facet joints prevent spinal damage and even if a spine is twisted to breaking point, an almost inconceivable physiological situation, it still does not produce a disc protrusion or prolapse. Indeed, if a disc is incised with a scalpel right through the annulus into the nucleus, so that it could well be envisaged that the nuclear material would extrude and the spine is loaded again to failure, no nuclear protrusion or extrusion occurs. Instead the vertebral bodies fracture again. Should a spine be flexed forward to failure, it does so by tearing the posterior ligamentous support of the spine or by fracturing the laminae and again does not produce a slipped disc. In an effort to try and produce a sudden disc prolapse, spines have been loaded to failure in multiple directions of load application with loads beyond those which would be encountered during life; and in these experiments involving cadaver spines, again some evidence of disc failure was produced, but only in a minority of not significantly *degenerate* discs. Meanwhile, *in vivo*, disc herniation only occurs in association with appreciable disc degeneration.

In one particular cadaver model, not only were the muscles, ribs and other important stress absorbers removed prior to experimentation, but also the actual laminae (the bony arches of the back of each vertebra) were taken away before loading. Even then, discs could not be damaged unless the joints were flexed well beyond the normal physiological range and the loads were increased to about a ton! Surgeons of all specialties do like to see patients and operate upon them, and engineers in much the same way like to make things and break them. In short, what these engineers showed is that if you cut out a cadaver joint, take away its shock absorbers, flex it beyond normal, hit it with a ton weight, a few normal discs may protrude.

Dr James Smeathers has spent much of his professional life studying the biomechanics of discs and was a colleague in the distinguished Rheumatism Research Unit in Leeds before taking on more senior academic challenges in the Antipodes. He wrote a very readable review article nicely entitled *Shocking news for discs*,[1] and in the first few paragraphs pointed out that orthopaedic surgeons, amongst others, commonly refer to intervertebral discs as *shock absorbers* and such statements still appear in orthopaedic textbooks despite the fact that there is not one iota of evidence to support such a notion. He demonstrated that as normal people move about, more than 80% of the load is taken by the legs and only about 16% by the spine and this is dealt with by the ligaments, muscles and vertebrae, and not by the discs. The discs are, therefore, not shock absorbers, but rather are a part of the spinal joint (mobile link), which in moving allows the ligaments to stretch and absorb the energy.

Smeathers also pointed out the very unfavourable energy considerations in the spontaneously occurring model of a spine devoid of all movement, the patient with *ankylosing spondylitis*. In this inflammatory arthritis of the spine, the disease leads to calcification and ossification of the various spinal ligaments and joints, such that no movement whatever occurs. The discs, of course, are spacers between the vertebrae, thus, allowing the spine to enjoy its great range of motion, and because loss of spinal movement cannot allow the ligaments and muscles to absorb the relevant energy, even something as seemingly low energy as putting one's heel to the ground in walking can for the ankylosing spondylitis patient result in a spinal fracture. He nicely paraphrased the notion that intervertebral discs are not shock absorbers by saying that if they were then *"there would be a one to two degree Celsius temperature rise every two or three seconds"* during life or to put it another way you would boil over running the hundred metres!

Smeathers

Intervertebral discs are spacers; they are not shock absorbers; they facilitate movement; they do not absorb energy.

Dr Michael Adams has done more than most to investigate the mechanical function of the intervertebral disc, particularly, as regards cadaver joint experimentation; and this distinguished bioengineer's recent review article[2] with his colleague Dr Dolan ought to be compulsory reading along with Smeathers' paper. He summarised a lot of work over the past two decades and concluded *"the notion that disc damage can be caused directly by compressive loading has been thoroughly disproved; compressive overload always affects the adjacent vertebral body even if the forces are applied repetitively or if the lamellae of the inner postero-lateral annulus are sectioned prior to loading"*.

This is not just a matter of considerable biomechanical interest, but utterly disproves the not uncommonly held belief, that annular tears can lead to subsequent disc prolapses. Dr Adams continued *"torsional loading damages the lumbar apophyseal joints (facet joints) long before the disc regardless of the precise orientation of the articular surfaces. If the apophyseal joints are removed then torsion eventually causes the lamellae of the annulus to separate circumferentially at about 10 to 20 degrees but without the formation of radial fissures or displacement of the nucleus pulposus"*. In effect, what Adams is saying is that the intervertebral discs are biomechanically, and thus traumatically, inviolate. That intervertebral discs are the strongest structures in the human spine is in no way surprising when one considers their form and structure (Fig. 4.8). The annulus, which is the fibrous surround of the disc and is effectively its ligament, is composed of immensely strong collagen fibres, which are gathered together into fibrous bundles, which undergo considerable interweaving and plaiting maximising their structural stability and resilience. Then to even further increase strength, as if that were necessary, the construct is then laminated.

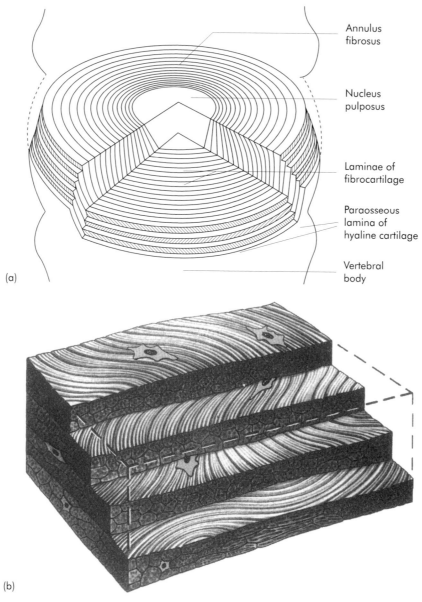

(a)

(b)

Fig. 4.8 (a) The main structural features of an intervertebral disc. For clarity, the number of fibrocartilaginous laminae has been greatly reduced, since they are in fact of microscopic dimensions. Note the alternating obliquity of collagen fascicles in adjacent laminae greatly strengthening the construct. (b) The arrangement of collagen fibres in ligament from Gray's anatomy. The direction of fibres is related to the stresses they undergo, but there is considerable interweaving of fibrous bundles, which greatly increases their structural stability and resilience. From Gray's Anatomy (1989). Eds Williams PL, Warnick R, Dyson M, Bannister LH. Thirty-Seventh Edition. Churchill Livingstone. Edinburgh & London.

Importantly, Adams went on to state *"discs that prolapse most easily in the laboratory are from the lower lumbar spine of cadavers aged under 50 years and it is interesting to note that these discs do not show any gross signs of degeneration. On the contrary, severely degenerated discs cannot be made to prolapse presumably because the nucleus is too fibrous to exert a hydrostatic pressure on the annulus"*. In other words, normal discs can give a bit even in these grossly unphysiological laboratory conditions, but degenerate ones cannot because quite simply they are too stiff. This kicks into touch the other oft-quoted assertion about disc hernias in relation to trauma that the degenerate annulus acts like a toothpaste tube and under load can squeeze out some nuclear material (toothpaste) when, in fact, precisely the *opposite* is the situation.

Adams

Intervertebral discs are inviolate to compressive and torsional forces. Degenerate discs are too stiff to be squeezed.

It can be seen, therefore, that for the sort of injuries that *experts* find themselves writing medical reports about and giving evidence in court about the effect on the intervertebral disc, it is abundantly clear no disc damage occurs with these sorts of fairly low-energy events. Even if that is accepted, it is often asserted that with very high-energy injuries, sufficient to damage the spine's natural shock absorbers, the disc is open to insult. But is there any evidence that this happens in real life or indeed to the degenerate disc? We certainly have not seen it ourselves in more than a quarter of a century and we staff a busy regional and supra-regional Spinal Treatment Centre. We were, therefore, not at all surprised by a recent publication from Holland by Prof. Verbout, who MRI scanned 63 patients, who had sustained serious fractures or fracture–dislocations of their thoraco-lumbar spine between 18 months and 5 years after the injury in question.[3] He found precious little evidence of intervertebral disc damage or degeneration at the site of injury and certainly not at adjacent sites, where huge loads would necessarily have had to be applied. He concluded that even when the shock absorbers are effectively broken and functionless, the intervertebral disc is still inviolate.

Verbout

In our study, lack of consistent MRI signal changes after a major traumatic event to the motion segment does not support the idea of a traumatic origin to degenerative disc disease.

Clinically, patients with disc hernias can present *acutely* with severe sciatica and/or indeed acute and severe neurological loss. The neurological loss can be as compelling as an acute cauda equina syndrome with loss of bowel and bladder function and perineal sensory loss; it can be less compelling but equally important in the form of, say, a drop foot with inability to extend the toes or foot in accordance with a complete L5 nerve root lesion. Surgeons have to operate within a matter of hours to give the patient the best recovery chance. These, of course, are not *acute* disc prolapses, but rather disc prolapses that have presented clinically and symptomatically in an acute fashion. Surgeons never see any evidence of trauma, when they operate on disc lesions even when they are supposedly acute. We would certainly expect to see some evidence of local bleeding as the degenerate discs' surrounding envelope is richly vascular. Not only do we not see any structural damage and bleeding from the muscles, ligaments and bones locally, but nothing at all from the disc itself. Then we very often send our disc fragments excised at surgery for histological examination, and there is never any evidence of trauma either recent in terms of blood staining or remote in terms of blood products (haemosiderin), just pure and simple degeneration (Fig. 4.5). But we can see signs of neovascularisation (new blood vessels growing). This sign is *diagnostic* of chronicity. Therefore, on clinical, pathological and biomechanical grounds, there is no substance at all for the notion that trauma in any way affects disc herniation which is, rather, part and parcel of the natural and constitutional process of degeneration, which is very much under genetic control.

Before looking at the question of MRI scanning in medico-legal practice and the evidence against any association between disc degeneration and trauma, we should summarise some of the very interesting and more recent epidemiological surveys concerning MRI scanning of volunteers. Battié and his group have looked at the Finnish identical twin cohort in a number of regards including MRI scanning.[4] They first published MRI scan results of 40 males (20 identical twin pairs) and showed a remarkable degree of correspondence of the site of degenerative changes throughout the twins' spines. For instance, we generally see evidence of degenerative change in cervical, thoracic and lumbar regions and this would be scattered about at relative random in the population at large. The twins had identical levels in the spine of degenerative change, for instance one pair might have C5/6 and C6/7 disease in association with lumbar L4/5 disease, whereas another pair of twins might have C6/7 disease with lumbar L3/4 disease, etc. It was abundantly clear to Battié and his colleagues that what was being looked at was a marked genetic influence and this, of course, warranted further investigation.

They then looked at 115 male identical twin pairs, who were assessed by MRI scanning, but also with an in-depth interview concerned with physical lifestyle, injuries and symptoms, and put the twins into two separate discordant groups (heavy work, twisting and bending, weight lifting, back "injuries", etc. versus the opposite). There was no difference in the degree or severity of the degenerative process indicating that the physical environment has little or no part to play.

Battié

The present study findings suggest that disc degeneration may be explained primarily by genetic influences … the particular environmental factors studied, which have been among those most widely suspected of accelerat-ing disc degeneration had very modest effects … and did not reach statistical significance in the lower lumbar region.

Then they went on to look at the effects of endurance exercise in 22 discordant twin pairs again MRI scanned. There was somewhat of a trend for lower thoracic disc degeneration to be reflected with more power sport involvement, but no trends whatever in terms of degeneration in the lower lumbar spine which, of course, is where we see our clinical disc hernias.

Meanwhile, the literature is replete with single case reports; and in 1996, there was a nice case study of a girl of 12 who developed backache and sciatica of such severity that surgery was contemplated and an MRI scan was carried out.[5] This showed multi-level lumbar disc degeneration and a big hernia at one level, but fortunately her symptoms settled and she did not require surgery. Her identical twin sister kindly volunteered for an MRI scan and basically the scans of the twin sisters could be freely interchanged because they showed exactly the same appearances. Studies trying to relate radiological changes in the spine to different occupations have very importantly ignored heredity as a confounding variable and to assume that certain occupations do not run in families and, therefore, a comparison between two occupations is not a comparison between two inheritances is fallacious to the point of being unacceptable. Statements such as "all the men in our family have worked in the pits since the 1800s when the pits first opened" and "my father and grandfather were also doctors" are very common and show how heredity and occupation go hand in hand. Furthermore, going back to some of the pre-MRI plain film investigations concerning different occupations what was not differentiated was the true process of degenerative change in the spine from the *physiology of life*. For true degeneration of a joint, you need to have joint space narrowing, marginal new bone formation (osteophytes) and subchondral sclerosis (thickening of the ends of the vertebrae on each side of the disc). Several studies have shown more osteophytes with a more physical life on this planet; but in the absence of concomitant joint space narrowing and subchondral sclerosis, such spurs of bone are where ligaments are inserted and, thus, these new spurs of bone have been formed by ligamentous traction on the vertebral edges. This is the physiology of life (Fig. 4.9) and not degeneration, which, like cancer or rheumatoid arthritis, is a disease and not a traumatic disorder.

Of course we know that personal injury claims for disc damage due to "trauma" continue apace and we know that literature is often quoted in support but is the opinion that trauma is in any way causative responsible and is the literature underpinning it valid. There are a number of such publications that don't meet the mark but one that is often quoted and relied upon in medical reports is that by the distinguished North American Epidemiologist Jennifer Kelsey.[6] In 1984 she published a paper entitled "An Epidemiological Study of Lifting and Twisting on the Job and Risks for Acute Prolapsed Lumbar Intervertebral

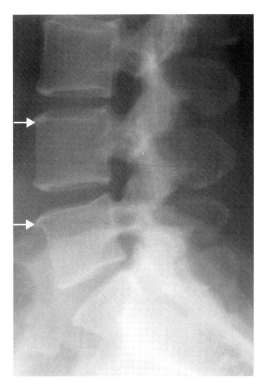

Fig. 4.9   X-ray of the lumbar spine showing marginal spurs of new bone formation. This is not degeneration; this is the physiology of life.

Disc" in which her message was that there was an up to six times higher incidence of acute prolapsed lumbar disc in those involved with lifting and twisting compared to controls. This paper is often referred to in review articles in support of the notion that there is a relationship between trauma and disc prolapse (e.g. reference 2 at the end of this chapter). The basic problem with this paper is not the impeccable methodology but the substrate. Cases were matched with controls "without known disc prolapse". The cases were collected between 1979 and 1981 and comprised 325 so-called cases of prolapsed lumbar intervertebral discs. The cases were divided into three categories according to strength of diagnosis – (1) surgical cases; (2) probable cases; (3) possible cases.

The surgical cases had a disc hernia identified at surgery but the rationale behind surgery was based upon either ordinary plain films (which have no diagnostic capability for disc prolapse) or myelography (prevalent as an investigation at the time but a crude diagnostic index). It is not clear how many of the definite surgical cases had confirmatory myelography but only a proportion.

Meanwhile in the 99 *probable* cases only 4 underwent surgery and the rest were diagnosed clinically with sciatica. In the *possible* cases only a complaint of thigh or leg pain was sufficient. Of course none of the controls had any form of imaging at all. Yes – a nice paper as regards epidemiological method; no – not helpful in terms of answering the question that the title addressed. In view of the enormous increase in our knowledge base about this subject and in particular MRI scanning, it is no longer acceptable to rely upon this sort of publication. The last two decades have seen an overwhelming amount of evidence that physical activities are irrelevant and one can go no further than references 8 and 12 at the end of this chapter to determine why.

Fraser's[7] group in Adelaide have attempted to relate trauma to disc degeneration in a number of ways. By openly incising through the annulus with a scalpel in sheep (thus exposing the inside of the disc to the outside world) they noted, not surprisingly, that blood vessels and other tissue gained entry and invaded the disc to produce pathological changes which they likened to degeneration. Of course in the human situation full thickness tears only occur in association with advanced stages of degeneration of which indeed they are a part, whereas, up until this end-stage, annular tears are not full thickness as Figure 4.4 clearly demonstrates.

To further their hypothesis they looked at cadaver discs and noted three types of annular tear, peripheral (parallel to the disc), circumferential (in the vertical axis of the disc) and radiating (parallel or oblique to the disc). The discs were excised from 27 post-mortem spines and in each spine all 5 lumbar discs were studied (L1/2 down to L5/S1). Peripheral lesions looked to them histologically more like trauma than degeneration. They thought that these peripheral lesions may "influence and accelerate the degeneration of the intervertebral disc, and play a part in producing discogenic pain". Of course the question of pain is highly speculative as these were cadaver specimens but 90% of disc degeneration and herniation in the lumbar spine occurs at the bottom two levels, L4/5 and L5/S1. These peripheral lesions were scattered throughout the lumbar spine and if they were to exert any aetiological or accelerating effect then degenerative change ought to be equally scattered throughout the lumbar spine and not focussed at the bottom two levels. That the bottom two levels are greatly over-represented indicates that this degenerative process is independent of peripheral lesions and accords with a natural, constitutional and essentially genetic process.

Meanwhile their more significant radial tears were always associated with, and were part and parcel of, "more advanced degeneration, forming clefts which radiated from the nucleus to the outer annulus". Not surprisingly half of all radial tears were at the L5/S1 level.

The last decade since these publications has however seen a considerable amount of epidemiological and MRI data, particularly that concerning heredity, that very considerably relegates the spine's physical environment.

Furthermore, the term *back injury* needs to be clearly defined with many individuals doing such things as yoga exercises, jogging, marathon running, recreational dancing and lifting something up; these must be regarded as activities of daily living and not discrete injuries in any causal relationship sense. Such histories of physical happenings occur in the population at large. If one does not accept the relevant literature about the lack of a relationship between *trauma* and disc degeneration/ herniation, and if one ignores the compelling identical twin studies, is it still acceptable to "guestimate" that intervertebral disc hernia patients commonly present after injury? Yes, if one recorded each of one's personal clinical cases as regards factors leading up to clinical presentation, document them *prospectively* and then analyse them. The late *Arthur Naylor* did just that and found that a physical event preceded clinical presentation in only 12–14% of his cases; moreover, those physical events were not all "injuries".[8] These figures suggest that there may in fact be a negative correlation rather than a positive one between the physical environment and clinical presentation. Naylor was the doyen of British lumbar spine surgery and two or three decades ago was the leading figure in British spinal research as regards lumbar intervertebral disc degeneration.

His chapter on lumbar disc disease in 1990 was probably the best stand-alone review of the subject in the English literature at that time.

In our centre, we carry out 2500 MRI scans of the spine each year, and have been unable to find a visible difference in the MRI appearance of a symptomatic from a non-symptomatic degenerated and/or herniated disc. We have not seen a difference in the appearance of a disc hernia, which is demonstrated in a patient who gives a history of injury from a patient who does not give a history of injury. We have not found an abnormality on MRI scanning or any other form of radiological investigation, which allows us to say that a disc hernia was of immediately recent onset, or was several months old, or was less than a-year old or was 2- rather than 3-years old or 3- rather than 4-years old. We have some confidence in stating that a disc hernia is 10- or 15-years old, and we are unable to say if an MRI abnormality of degeneration and/or herniation is symptomatic or will become symptomatic and if so when. We also have patients who have been listed for discectomy on the basis of matching symptoms, signs and MRI appearances who have become symptom-free prior to admission, but still have exactly the same disc prolapse with nerve root compression when the MRI scan has been repeated.

The tissues surrounding the degenerate disc are vascular, and in patients who have a spinal dislocation through a spinal joint, where the annulus is known to be torn, haemorrhage is a feature on every MRI scan (Fig. 4.10). If annular tears (HIZs) were traumatic events (similar to a dislocation although less severe), then we should anticipate seeing haemorrhage associated with these tears albeit in smaller quantities. Although MRI scanning is very sensitive to haemorrhage, we have neither seen such haemorrhages associated with a disc hernia nor have we ever seen haemorrhage or haemosiderin mentioned in the literature which describes the MRI findings of disc herniation.

No one has been able to relate annular tears to a history of injury or to pathological findings of injury, and these so-called tears are no different from fissures, which are a feature of disc degeneration[9] (Fig. 4.5). It is important to note that these HIZs are invariably demarcated posteriorly by a membrane; and if

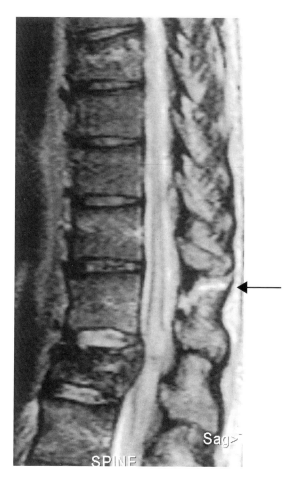

Fig. 4.10 Sagittal MRI section showing bleeding (white signal-arrowed) in association with a fracture–dislocation of the spine.

they were traumatic disruptions to the posterior annulus, it would be astonishing to see that the thin peripheral membrane did not also tear (Fig. 4.4). Such traumatic disruption does occur with dislocation and does not leave thin layers with the posterior annular fibres in tact.

We have never come across an article in the literature of the English-speaking world which indicates that the radiological signs of injury are seen associated with disc herniation. The MRI experience of disc herniation is now immense; and in that immense experience, there has been no example of lumbar disc herniation being caused by non-disruptive trauma. It is long past time that radiologists anyway, if not spinal surgeons, accept that there is no evidence of an association between the two and that it requires great imagination to suggest otherwise. It is now well known that disc degeneration is a hereditary condition with such strong heritability that a single gene is most likely to be the cause. Dutch epidemiologists have clearly demonstrated in meta-analysis reviews of the X-ray literature that no firm evidence exists for the presence of a number of plain X-ray findings and non-specific back pain and these findings would include: *slight degeneration, advanced disc degeneration, spondylosis, spondylolisthesis, spina bifida, transitional vertebrae, Scheuermann's disease,* as almost half of the individuals with these various conditions do not have back pain.[10]

The sensitivity of MRI scanning makes this investigation even less predictive to the point where MRI scanning should not be performed for the purposes of personal injury litigation. The results of the investigation are irrelevant since the finding of disc degeneration and/or herniation cannot be causally related to symptoms, prognosis, cause, time of onset of the abnormality (if one is present) or its relevance to the injury in question. The medical prognostication of a litigant is a clinical matter, MRI has no place. The possible findings on MRI scanning of a personal injury litigant are a negative or normal examination, one or more levels of degeneration, one or more disc hernias. A negative or normal examination does not indicate that there is no organic cause for the individual's complaints and a normal MRI scan does not have a better prognosis than an MRI that shows degeneration and/or herniation. Degeneration and/or herniation are extremely common in the asymptomatic general population, and the MRI findings in these individuals are identical to those found in a claimant. The claimant will argue that the abnormality was caused or made worse by the injury in question, and the defence will counter that none of the findings is caused by injury or is made worse by injury. Carrying out the MRI scan will increase the argument and the extent of the action, and we certainly have never known an MRI scan to settle an argument in personal litigation, and it has been our invariable experience that the introduction of an MRI scan increases the arguments and the expense of the action. It is not all that unusual in our experience for an MRI scan to be the sole force preventing resolution and driving a trial. Moreover, MRI scanning is hazardous to the litigant because after the trial he will still have his pain and will have a judicial decision, which *proved* that the abnormality shown by the MRI was the cause of his pain.

Armed with this *abnormal* MRI scan and persisting pain, the litigant will find a surgeon who will operate on his back. This is the beginning of the long slippery slope into the total incapacity of post-laminectomy failure. There is absolutely no possibility that an individual who has been litigating for at least 5 years and suffering from back pain all the while will have his back pain made better by surgery. It is almost a certainty that his back pain will be made worse.

Finally as regards degenerative disc disease and its aetiology and natural history, there is the frequently termed expression *acceleration*. There are semantic, medical and legal implications concerning this word. Acceleration might suggest the hastening of a pathological process such as degenerative disc disease, or it may be intended to mean that an injury has provoked symptoms from a pre-existing degenerative condition, or it may mean that the natural history of degenerative disc disease has been accelerated as a result of injury. Orthopaedic surgeons have known for decades if not centuries what the effect of trauma on joints means. There are two kinds of *degenerative disease* – primary and secondary. The lady in Figure 2.6 has primary hip arthritis. This is a genetic, natural and constitutional process very similar to degenerative spinal disease and occurs more in females because they are much more vulnerable genetically than men to wear and tear arthritis. Trauma has had nothing whatever to do with this condition pathologically. Meanwhile secondary arthritis is attributable to some pre-existing disease or deformity of the joint or trauma sufficient to produce a fracture or dislocation of the joint. Thus, patients who have had hip disease in childhood, for example congenital hip dislocation or Perthes' disease (Fig. 4.11), have developed a hip shape which is not symmetrical and thus promotes the development of early secondary osteoarthritis. Thus one of these childhood conditions can produce arthritis in their twenties and thirties whereas primary arthritis would tend to occur in the fifties or sixties.

The effect of trauma on joints is well known. Front seat passengers in high speed head-on road traffic accidents are very prone to suffer the injury of a fracture–dislocation of the hip

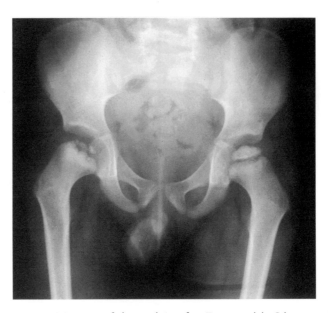

Fig. 4.11   AP view of the pelvis of a 7 year old. Observe that the head of the femur (the ball of the ball and socket) on the right side has not developed properly, is small and fragmented. This is Perthes' disease. If it remains deformed it will produce early secondary arthritis.

joint. The patient sits with hips and knees flexed to 90 degrees and on impact the thighbone is driven backwards by contact with the dashboard and fractures through the socket in the pelvis to produce a nasty fracture–dislocation. One of the most dreaded complications of such an injury, even when the parts are put together anatomically, is the development of early secondary arthritis (Fig. 4.12). This can occur within a matter of a few years unlike primary arthritis which occurs over many decades. However if the road traffic accident had energy just under that required to produce a fracture–dislocation, i.e. the hip joint didn't sustain any structural failure, then there is no initiation of arthritis in a normal joint, nor acceleration of arthritis in an already arthritic joint. This is why marathon runners have even less hip arthritis than secretaries because it is not the repetitive pounding of a normal hip joint that matters, rather whether one is more inclined to primary generalised arthritis as a female. Thus it is that the necessary and crucial ingredient in the process of initiation or acceleration is primary structural damage to the joint concerned. Thus in the

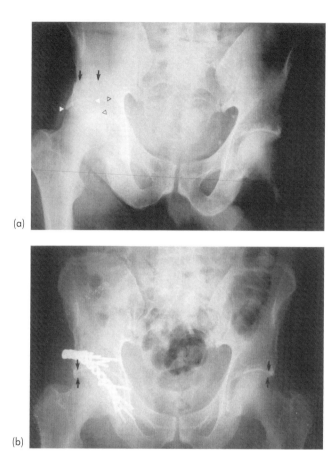

Fig. 4.12 (a) AP X-ray of the pelvis showing a nasty fracture–dislocation of the right hip hoint. The dislocation has been reduced and the broken socket can clearly be seen. A large fragment of socket (black arrows and white arrowheads) has displaced sideways and there are other small socket fragments (hollow arrowheads). (Patient of Mr Peter Giannoudis.) (b) In an effort to put the socket fragments together as accurately as possible a plate and screws have been inserted. An almost anatomical reduction has been achieved, and the hip joint space (between ball and socket) is as good as the contralateral normal side (arrows).

fracture–dislocation of the spine there are not only initial problems that have to be dealt with but also because a joint has been significantly structurally damaged there certainly is a risk of early secondary osteoarthritis (Fig. 2.7). If the energies are insufficient to cause structural failure, as in the vast majority

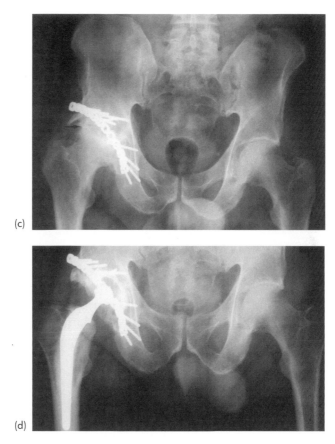

(c)

(d)

Fig. 4.12 (c) Notwithstanding within two years there was the development of very severe degenerative arthritis with considerable joint space narrowing (arrow), sclerosis and marginal osteophytes formation. Compare this appearance with the normal left hip and the normal right hip in Figure 2.6a. (d) Like the lady in Figure 2.6 the arthritis has been dealt with by a Charnley total hip replacement.

of back injuries, then no pathological process has been generated to account for long-term disability.

The natural history of primary arthritis of the hip is that, say, in the early fifties when it starts, there is the occasional twinge of groin pain with a fairly severe physical activity such as digging, and there would be an appreciable symptom-free interval before the next episode of discomfort. Then as time goes on the symptom-free intervals reduce while the physical intensity of the required insult also reduces until years or decades later the patient has severe hip joint symptoms on a daily basis with normal activities of daily living.

Although degenerative spinal disease is not strictly comparable to hip arthritis, in that severe degenerative disease on spine X-rays or scans may be entirely symptom-free, nonetheless the same argument is often used about the effects of trauma on pre-existing spinal degeneration. Therefore, yes, if you have a nasty fracture or dislocation of the spine, you can initiate degenerative change in a normal spine or accelerate any pre-existing degenerative change before the injury and we would champion your cause. No – if you have an injury that does not cause structural failure to the spine then it certainly does not accelerate the underlying pathological process of degeneration.

If in the general practitioner records there are ever more frequent entries of low back pain occurring initially relatively infrequently latterly more frequently with normal activities then this would be the natural history of degenerative spinal disease. There is no pathological basis to support the notion that someone with no past history suddenly develops symptoms from pre-existing degenerative spinal disease and is disabled thereafter. It is simply not the natural history of degenerative disease. Thus the notion that an individual, particularly a young person, could sustain a soft tissue lumbar strain and then have long-term disability attributed to the provocation of symptoms from pre-existing MRI changes is quite untenable. Therefore an opinion to be put forward that, had the individual concerned not had the injury, a soft tissue ligamentous strain with no injury to discs or joints, they would have been able to carry on working for a further ten years has simply no organic basis. Alternatively if the moving of a piece of furniture was the injury in question then a comparable force must be applied to the spine in any event within a matter of days as such a task would be regarded as being routine.

Sub-structural failure injury of a joint can certainly lead to a very painful musculo-ligamentous strain. As no structural damage to the joint occurs then there is no pathological process generated to account for long-term disability. Symptoms can be very painful to begin with but are relatively short-lived in a matter of weeks or months. Such injuries would have no effect on the status of the underlying joint. It is simply not the natural history of degenerative disease of any joint to be provoked into severe and long-term disability, without a significant past history, without structural damage to that joint. If the individual's back is for whatever reason that vulnerable then a comparable "injury" would occur in any event in a relatively short timeframe.

CLINICAL FEATURES

Now looking at the clinical features of lumbar disc hernia-tion,[11] we recall that the PLL directs the hernia postero-laterally (Fig. 4.6) just where the nerve root is. Again for genetic reasons, it tends to be the bottom two discs that are affected by this natural process of degeneration and these are the L4/5 and the L5/S1 discs. Together, they account for more than 90% of lumbar disc hernias with nearly all the remainder being at the level above, the L3/4 level. It is exceptional for disc herniation to occur higher up in the lumbar spine. Therefore, for practical purposes, one needs to consider what happens at the L3/4, L4/5 and L5/S1 intervertebral disc levels. It is the L4 nerve root, which crosses the L3/4 disc and can be affected by an L3/4 disc hernia. The L5 nerve root crosses the L4/5 disc and the S1 root crosses the L5/S1 disc, and so these roots can be affected by disc hernias at these levels, respectively (Fig. 4.13).

Back pain localised to the mid-lumbar level might suggest an L3/4 disc problem in contrast to lumbo-sacral localised pain, which might suggest an L5/S1 disc hernia, but the level of the perceived back pain is nowhere near precise enough to identify levels. Rather it is the distribution of neurological involvement that matters here. Each spinal nerve root is like a branch of a tree, and if something is irritating or compressing the branch as it exits from the trunk of the tree, then symptoms can be felt anywhere in the distribution of that branch from just where it leaves the main tree trunk right out to the terminal twigs. Therefore, nerve root symptoms can be felt right out to the terminal distribution of the finer branches of that nerve root. These distributions are well known to spinal surgeons, who in turn use the distribution of symptoms to localise the problem to a particular spinal level. Due to the predictability of the distribution of the L4, L5 and S1 nerve roots, the localisation of levels can be a very precise matter. Thus, L4 nerve root pain tends to be felt in the groin, the anterior thigh, and the front and inside of the leg down to the ankle on the inside. L5 nerve root pain can be felt in

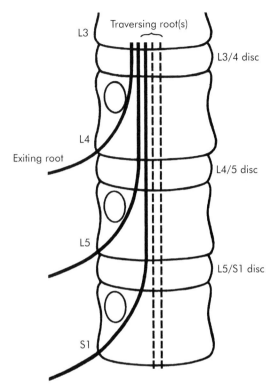

Fig. 4.13　The L4 nerve root crosses the L3/4 disc, the L5 nerve root crosses the L4/5 disc and the S1 root crosses the L5/S1 disc.

the buttock, the back and side of the thigh, the side of the calf, and then it tends to go across towards the big toe on the dorsum (upper) of the foot. S1 root pain can be felt in the buttock, the back of the thigh, the back of the calf to the heel, the sole of the foot and the lesser toes (Fig. 2.14). A feature common to L4, L5 and S1 root pain is that it goes *below* the knee. Indeed, true sciatica *must* go below the knee.

Root distributions

- L4 – front of shin to inside of ankle
- L5 – side of leg below knee towards big toe
- S1 – back of calf to heel and sole of foot to lesser toes

The character of *radicular* (nerve root) pain is also very important here. It tends to be a shooting, severe, electrical type of pain of completely different quality from *referred* back pain. Furthermore, it must go below the knee; and in this way, it can be differentiated from the associated back pain. Back pain can radiate as far as buttock and even thigh but not below the knee and, secondly, referred pain from the back is of the same quality as the back pain generally being rather dull and mechanical.

Therefore, if a patient attends the doctor with low-back pain with radiation to buttock and upper thigh, then this is non-specific low-back pain and may be coming from a degenerate disc that is bulging; but as there are no localising neurological features, its precise location and cause cannot be determined nor for that matter is it particularly important at least from the surgical point of view because, as mentioned previously, surgery for disc problems is addressed to the neurological consequences and not to the back pain itself. Such symptoms would tend to settle with the passage of time and appropriate supportive therapy.

With low-back pain of any cause, but with discogenic pain in particular, the paraspinal muscles that run down the back of the spine very often go into a degree of protective spasm in an attempt to immobilise the level involved and, therefore, in some way protect it. This spasm produces two clinical features – a reduction in movements of the spine because the muscles would not relax to allow movement to occur and, secondly, flattening of the normal hollow behind the lumbar spine (lordosis). The muscle spasm pulls the back of the spine backwards, and so on examination, some flattening of the lumbar lordosis and reduced movements are to be expected. These signs are not specific for a disc problem at any particular level or of any particular clinical significance, rather they indicate a painful back. If the youngish adult reports to the doctor with a history of recent onset low-back pain in association with a severe shooting electrical-type pain down the back of the right thigh, back of the calf to the sole of the foot and to the lesser toes, then the doctor can confidently diagnose a right-sided L5/S1 disc prolapse – a big enough disc hernia to irritate the transiting nerve root, which at the L5/S1 level is the S1 nerve root. If the youngish adult reported a nasty electrical toothache in the left leg which was felt in the buttock, the back and outside of the thigh and the outside of the calf to the big toe, then one can confidently diagnose a left L4/5 disc prolapse. Whether a loose piece of disc is present (sequestration) or there is a simple prolapse is something seen on subsequent scanning and is of no material consequence to the situation at least at this stage.

When we lie down supine our leg, straight at the knee, can usually be passively raised to about 90°. As the nerve roots move through their canals during a straight leg raise (SLR), they might be abraded if they are in contact with a disc hernia and, therefore, SLR is less than normal. This is the basis of the SLR test (Figs 4.14a, b and 4.14c, d). It is important that this SLR reduction has to be caused by the same radicular pain the patient mentioned in the history and not, for instance, a non-specific feature, such as low-back pain. Thus, an SLR of only 20° before a sciatic pain was produced in the leg would be indicative of a potentially more serious disc problem than one, where SLR was only terminally reduced at, say 70°. And indeed the difference in SLR over time is a useful index as regards the natural history of the intervertebral disc problem, that is, getting better or getting worse; you treat patients and not scans.

We mentioned that nerve roots can be irritated or compressed and the clinician now wants to know whether the patient we have described presenting with right S1 root pain or left L5 root pain does have objective evidence of interference with the function of that root. What is important here is objective evidence rather than subjective evidence. For instance, a change in the reflexes or obvious muscle weakness with muscle wasting are much more important physical signs than, say, an area of slightly reduced sensation to pin prick. Fortunately, each of these nerve roots, L4, L5 and S1, does have very good objective neurological evidence of compression, and in the neurological assessment of the patient, these objective neurological signs should be specifically looked for. The L4 nerve root supplies the knee jerk, while the S1 nerve root supplies the ankle jerk. With the knees semi-flexed and relaxed over the examiner's forearm, the knee reflexes can be elicited. What matters is the symmetry between right and left sides. Some normal people have very brisk reflexes and some normal people have no reflexes at all. If, therefore, neither reflex can be elicited, then no information can be gained; but if one side is obviously suppressed compared to the other, then that is evidence of nerve root compression. The L4 nerve root also supplies the quadriceps muscle on the front of the thigh and, therefore, some degree of muscle wasting is sometimes seen with long-standing L4 nerve

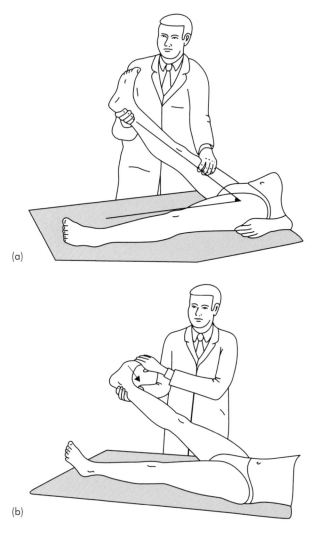

Fig. 4.14(a, b) *The three nerve root tension tests.* (a) SLR; this is positive if an SLR reproduces the patient's sciatica appreciably before 90°. (b) The sciatic stretch test (SST); if on an SLR sciatica is produced and then the leg is lowered a few degrees, and the leg pain stops the ankle is dorsi-flexed and the sciatic pain returns, this is a positive test.

root compression, but an actual reduction in power of that muscle's ability to straighten the knee is seldom demonstrable.

The ankle reflexes are similarly elicited with the knee semi-flexed and the ankle dorsiflexed and again it is inequality which is being looked for. An absent ankle reflex is very commonly

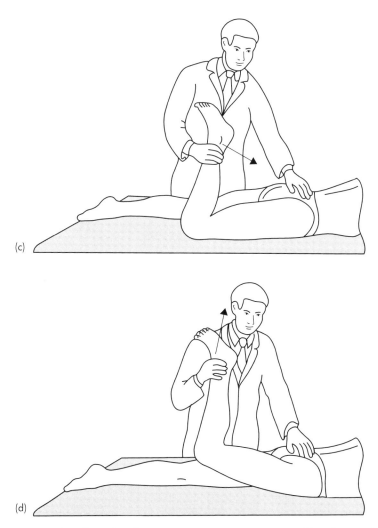

Fig. 4.14(c, d) *The three nerve root tension tests.* The femoral stretch test (FST); this is specifically for the L4 nerve root and when the knee is flexed and hip extended, and a sciatic pain is felt in the front of the thigh and inside of the leg, then this test is positive.

encountered with S1 nerve root compression. The L5 nerve root does not supply a reflex, but it does supply the muscle which extends or lift up the big toe (as well as the other toes and the foot as a whole). Any degree of L5 nerve root compression is demonstrable by a clear weakness of the power of lifting up the big toes towards the face against the examiner's hands. Should clear weakness be elicited, then it is important to look for and measure the calf circumferences at an equal distance down the calf from the knee. Any significant degree of muscle weakness ought to be accompanied by muscle wasting, otherwise it raises the possibility of inappropriate illness behaviour (see later).

- L4 nerve root – knee reflex
- L5 nerve root – power of toe extension
- S1 nerve root – ankle reflex

The following clinical scenarios might be helpful in appreciating what doctors, and spinal surgeons in particular, infer from clinical examination and changes in individual patients.

If we go back to our young adult who presented with a nasty shooting electrical-type pain in the buttock, posterior thigh, posterior calf to the sole of the foot and lesser toes of, say, 4 weeks duration, then we will want to examine the patient. We might find some flattening of the lumbar lordosis and forward spinal flexion reduced to half-normal as a consequence of the muscle spasm, but we want to know much more about the nerve root and in particular its function. SLR may be reduced to, say, 45° and the ankle reflex might be present. This would suggest that the nerve root is being irritated but not being compressed. Non-operative treatment should be prescribed starting perhaps with referral to a physiotherapist and for recalcitrant cases epidural or nerve root injections of a long-acting local anaesthetic and an anti-inflammatory drug. Surgical treatment should not be rushed into until non-operative treatment has been seen to fail or significant clinical deterioration has been observed. Alternatively, SLR may be 20° and the ankle reflex absent and this latter clinical situation would be regarded as more surgically relevant.

Similarly, the young adult that presented with features of an L4/5 disc prolapse with L5 nerve root irritation may have on examination SLR of 60° (the L5 nerve root moves less through its canal than the S1 nerve root on an SLR) and the power of extension of the big toe might be normal in which case we could infer that there was evidence of L5 nerve root irritation, but not compression. Again a course of non-operative therapy should be administered. If the patient was then given an appointment for 4 weeks time and we then found that SLR on the left side was down to 30° and that power of extension of the big toe was obviously less than on the other side we can infer that there is clear evidence of L5 nerve root compression, the clinical situation is deteriorating and action should be taken. Moreover, the L5 nerve root is much less robust than the S1 root and L5 muscle weakness is common, while S1 muscle weakness is rare. In addition, severe degrees of *drop foot* (inability to extend the foot and toes) often do not fully recover and, therefore, the threshold for prescribing L5 root decompression is much lower than for the S1 root.

At this time, *and not before*, radiological studies should be carried out and in this day and age, we are referring to MRI scanning.[12] The specific reason for requesting an MRI scan is to confirm that there is an intervertebral disc hernia at the level the surgeon thinks (e.g. L4/5 or L5/S1) and on the side he thinks (i.e. left or right) and that the rest of the spine is preferably pristine. In those circumstances, it is logical to consider surgical intervention. As something like 30% of 30-year olds, 50% of 50-year olds, etc. can be demonstrated to have a disc hernia of surgical significance on an MRI scan, yet are entirely symptom free, mismatches are more common than we would like. Indeed, Boos *et al.* compared the MRI scans of 43 patients with sciatica who underwent surgery for a disc hernia with 43 age and sex-matched controls who had *never* had sciatica or any back symptoms. While all the patients had a disc hernia on the scan, as many as 76% of the asymptomatic controls had a disc hernia on scanning.[13] Therefore, if the patient we suspect of having a right L5/S1 disc hernia with reduced SLR who is not improving with the passage of time or who is deteriorating in terms of the severity of the radicular pain, and we order an MRI scan and it reveals a left L4/5 disc prolapse and a very unimpressive appearance on the right side at the L5/S1 level, then surgery is *not indicated*. This sort of mismatch scenario occurs much more commonly than you might imagine, and hence, inappropriate surgical intervention is regrettably too often prescribed presumably because of the compelling scan appearances. However, one treats the patient and not the X-rays.

True sciatica

- Not improving ± neurological signs
- More leg than back symptoms
- Surgery decided upon
- Then scan

Another common MRI finding is that while for our patient with a very nice big and juicy right-sided L5/S1 disc hernia, there is also a similar disc hernia at the level above (i.e. the L4/5 level on the right side); yet, of course, there were no right L5 nerve root symptoms. Whatever else, this individual must *not* have the L4/5 disc hernia operated on as it is quite asymptomatic. This patient merely has a double dose of genetic degeneration. Again, treat the patient and not the scan. We were recently sent a patient, fortunately from outside the Yorkshire region, who had had an MRI scan for not particularly strict criteria and had evidence of black discs (degeneration) at L2/3, L3/4, L4/5 and L5/S1. All of these had been removed and the patient, not surprisingly, had even more back pain than to start with. The patient was referred with the question "Please can you help?"; of course, this was beyond surgical salvage.

Very importantly, because MRI scanning of the disc patient should only be carried out if surgery is deemed a reasonable option, then axiomatically MRI scanning should not be ordered by anyone else, but the operating surgeon. It should not be other health care professionals, who have these scans carried out for disc hernia patients. If a neurologist thinks that a spinal cord tumour might be present or the rheumatologist suspects a nasty arthritis such as ankylosing spondylitis then, fair enough; but if the patient has disc hernia symptoms, then they should refer the patient to the spinal surgeon (orthopaedic or neurosurgeon) first *before* the scan. While intervertebral disc hernias may well be within their clinical knowledge portfolio, the natural history of disc hernias, with and without surgery, the nuances of surgical intervention, particularly if it is repeat surgery, only belongs to the spinal surgeon. Therefore, if doctors other than spinal surgeons encounter disc patients, access to MRI scanning should not be granted. Rather the patient should be referred with a letter saying, for instance, this patient did have low-back pain until 3 weeks ago when a nasty L5 sciatica developed. There is weakness of extensor hallucis longus and I think the patient might be suitable for surgical intervention. Then the spinal surgeon can assess the matter, decide if surgery is a correct option, and order the relevant imaging technique.

Regrettably, we are more and more encountering individuals who have had MRI scans at the request of lawyers. In simple terms, there is absolutely no point in knowing what genetic hand the person was dealt unless there are clinically compelling reasons toward surgical intervention and if that is the situation, then it should be the experienced spinal surgeon who should be at the helm, not the neurologist or rheumatologist and certainly not the lay or legal community. The "first doctor" syndrome, where the patient believes what the *first* doctor tells them, is very important in this context. The "black disc" on the MRI scan is analogous to the Blind Pew* syndrome of labelling by MRI appearance. It is the patient that should be addressed, not just the scan.

As there is a trend for ever increasing the availability of MRI scanning right down to primary care colleagues our plea looks rather forlorn. For the person whose clinical condition is worsening in terms of increasingly more severe or frequent radicular pain, and particularly the one who has objective neurological abnormalities, surgery is a sensible way forward, but it needs to be set in its proper context.

TREATMENT OF DISC HERNIAS

Not surprisingly, with MRI scanning giving you your genetic spinal coding, patients' symptomatology and MRI scanning do not always match up. If, however, the clinical features do indicate one-level nerve root problems and the MRI scan matches, then one is moving towards a surgical solution. Surgery is still a long way away. There really is only one reason for urgent disc surgery and that is the patient with fulminating neurological dysfunction. At the L4/5 level, there is sometimes a huge posterior disc hernia despite the presence of the PLL. The lower lumbar and sacral nerve roots are squashed up into the top of the attic underneath the roof and the nerves to the bladder can be readily dysfunctioned (Fig. 4.15). This is the acute *cauda equina syndrome* and there tends to be, in association with bladder symptoms, severe shooting bilateral sciatic-type pains to the feet. This is the absolute surgical emergency. There is no room for procrastination and the patient should be admitted forthwith, examined immediately, and if MRI scanning is available,

---

*Remember Blind Pew in Treasure Island blaming all and sundry and lashing out blindly for the loss of the contents of Captain Flint's sea-chest.

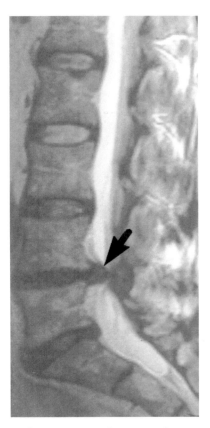

Fig. 4.15 Sagittal MRI section showing a huge L4/5 disc hernia almost completely blocking the spinal canal (arrow).

and it certainly should be if the patient has been referred to that particular hospital, then it should be carried out within a matter of half-an-hour to an hour. Then immediately thereafter, if the MRI scan has confirmed a huge L4/5 disc hernia, the patient should be taken to the operating room for discectomy and cauda equina decompression. In the *old days*, this would be done by a radical laminectomy (Fig. 3.5); in other words, removal of the roof of one or more houses, in the belief that this degree of destruction was required to produce adequate exposure so that the very big disc hernia could be delivered safely. Over the past 10 or more years, microdiscectomy techniques have become the gold standard, and it is perfectly possible using a microscope to approach the disc from one side and deliver disc material entirely safely without destroying the posterior spinal elements (Fig. 4.2). You certainly do not nowadays have to open the knee joint in a macro-fashion to deliver a big cartilage tear and nor do you have to do a radical laminectomy to deliver a large L4/5 posterior disc prolapse. Those who would say that they would do this non-microsurgically using spectacles with magnifying loupes, or even without, need to go that little bit further forward in their surgical development. It has happened in general surgery with laparoscopic abdominal techniques and it really should be more widely practised in spinal surgery. You only require a small hole to look down through a microscope and, of course, the lighting passes straight down the microscope, referred to as co-axial lighting, and combined with the great magnification of the microscope makes dissection between neurological and non-neurological structures a surgical delight. With a microdiscectomy, only three structures are incised – the overlying skin, the thoraco-lumbar fascia and the ligamentum flavum. Then the nerve root is identified and elevated with a nerve root retractor to allow the underlying disc to be delivered piecemeal (Fig. 4.2).

CAUDA EQUINA COMPRESSION

Cauda equina compression is a common focus for medical negligence suits, and perhaps here is the appropriate place to provide some further clinical detail.

Although nerve tissue is very delicate, it is forgiving for a while and it is this golden period that is crucial here. The brain is inside the rigid skull and the spinal cord and cauda equina are within the firm but less rigid spinal column. It is characteristic of the stroke patient to experience the *worst imaginable* headache before neurological dysfunction or collapse or whatever. Similarly, it takes time for pressure to build up on the cauda equina, or spinal cord, before neurological abnormalities occur. We have already mentioned the importance of an intact dural sleeve containing cerebro-spinal fluid under pressure to exert a hydrostatic beneficial effect on the contained nerve tissue, and we have already seen the disadvantage of a dural leak.

The literature on the subject of big L4/5 mid-line disc hernias causing cauda equina dysfunction is not particularly helpful, but no one would disagree with the assertion that the sooner decompression is carried out the better the result for the patient.

What really matters in terms of recovery is whether the degree of paralysis is complete or partial regardless of the duration of neurological abnormality. If the paralysis is incomplete, then surgical decompression can be expected to produce complete relief of neurological problems. If the degree of paralysis is complete, then decompression within the first 24 h can be expected to produce some neurological relief and this figure would approach 100%, if decompression was carried out in the first 8–12 h. Beyond 24 h, some degree of useful recovery might occur in occasional cases up to say 48 h. Therefore, it is virtually never too late to operate, particularly given the alternative of an asexual incontinent life sentence.

Now going back to routine disc surgery, unremitting sciatic pain plus or minus unfavourable neurological features is the surgical indication and, as mentioned previously, the gold standard is microdiscectomy. It has been said that progress in surgery is made by responsible clinical experimentation and the last two decades has seen the introduction of percutaneous and laser disc techniques. The protagonists vigorously pursued their beliefs, while the rest of the spinal world stood back to see if the results in sufficient numbers over sufficient time would make them add these techniques to their surgical armamentarium. It is difficult to understand why such techniques might work because the entire surgical issue is the removal of disc material pressing on the nerve root, not debulking the centre of the disc percutaneously either by sucking out disc material or vaporising it with a laser. Indeed, either of those techniques might be expected to make the outer annulus bulge even more. Perhaps, not surprisingly, randomised controlled trials have shown that percutaneous and laser techniques do not alter the natural history of a disc hernia and are not effective.[14,15]

One prospective randomised controlled trial of percutaneous discectomy had to be abandoned because the results were so poor,[16] and one prospective controlled trial of laser discectomy showed it was no better than an epidural injection[17] (local anaesthetic plus steroid injected around the relevant nerve root). Such techniques have been condemned by more than one international authority.[18,19]

Notwithstanding the excellent success rate with microdiscectomy, significant benefit is only for the first few years. Four to five years after surgery, there is no perceived benefit in terms of pain relief over patients treated non-surgically.[20] In other words, the 90% success rate is achieved non-operatively at 4–5 years. Of course, the patient with severe unremitting sciatica would find 4–5 years of agony to be quite unacceptable and would put themselves forward as surgical candidates. However, that is not the situation in the majority and a non-operative pain therapy strategy is well worth pursuing, at least to begin with. There is some evidence that with sciatica of beyond 6 months to a year duration, the results of surgical intervention are less good and, therefore, there is a time span within which surgical treatment should be carried out; unfortunately increased waiting lists and outpatient waiting times militate against achieving the best outcomes.

SPINAL STENOSIS

Whereas it is the L4/5 and L5/S1 discs which degenerate and herniate in the vast majority of patients, it is the L3/4 and L4/5 levels which tend to be involved in spinal stenosis. Again this is very much a genetic process and is much more common in females who are much more likely to be affected by *primary generalised osteoarthritis*.

This can affect the terminal joints in the fingers, the base joint of the thumb, the big toe metatarso-phalangeal joint, the hips, the knees, but particularly the lower neck and back. Whereas disc hernias bulge upwards through the ceiling into the attic spinal stenosis is effectively the sloping roof caving downwards and inwards into the attic.

This is because spinal stenosis is produced by osteoarthritis of the posterior facet joints. As with osteoarthritis in any joint, the articular hyaline cartilage self-destructs and the forces of life are taken on the nearby bone, which thickens in response. Thus, it might well be imagined that degenerative wear and tear means loss of substance, but it does actually mean increasing bone thickness (it is the cartilage that wears and not the bone). Therefore, osteoarthritis is the proliferative form of arthritis in contrast to inflammatory arthritides (such as rheumatoid disease), which are erosive and destructive. This degenerative process, rather like disc herniation, takes place over decades and indeed a somewhat longer time frame than disc herniation, and so patients tend to be appreciably older with spinal stenosis.

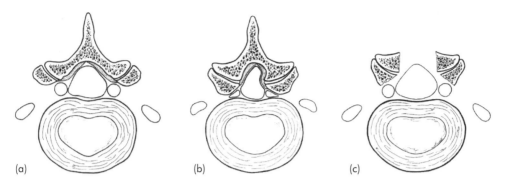

(a) (b) (c)

Fig. 4.16 Transverse sections of the lumbar spine. (a) The normal situation with a capacious canal. (b) Facet joint overgrowth in association with degenerative arthritis has grown in and produced a trefoil-shaped canal with both central and root canal stenosis. (c) After decompressive laminectomy and under-cutting facetectomy the central and root canals have been restored to their normal size.

Gradually, over these decades, the attic ever narrows making the space for the cauda equina ever smaller. As the posterior facet joints are about half-way down the sloping roof on each side, then the triangular attic becomes more and more trefoil shaped (Fig. 4.16). Thus, the volume of the attic steadily diminishes and if the bone thickening tends to affect the lower part of the roof on each side, then the canals through which the nerve roots exit from the spine are preferentially narrowed and this we call *lateral or root canal stenosis*. It is often extraordinary to see the amount of narrowing that can take place, often to a nearly complete or indeed complete block (i.e. there appears to be no space in the attic at all) and yet patients may have very little in the way of objective neurological dysfunction (Fig. 4.17). Nerve tissue is certainly forgiving, if it is compressed over many years. Indeed, sometimes the *block* can be present over two or more levels without there being much, or indeed any, neurological dysfunction.

There are three main methods of clinical presentation for patients with spinal stenosis – non-specific back pain (because of the facet joint arthritis), spinal claudication (cramps and tiredness in the legs which tend to be exercise-related) from central canal narrowing, and sciatic-type leg pains (although this third mode of presentation is the least common) from nerve root irritation. Despite the appearance of gross arthritis on the X-rays, these patients tend to have an apparently full range of spinal motion, although it may well be that much of it comes

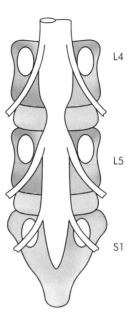

L4

L5

S1

Fig. 4.17   Diagram to show what stenosis does to the cauda equina. Sometimes there is no space at all for the nerve roots.

from the hip joints. This is because the back is much less irritable in degenerative arthritis than it is with a big disc prolapse and there is much less muscle spasm to impair motion. There is seldom any objective neurological change in terms of reduced sensation, or power, or reflex alteration.

However, the fourth dimension, time, is important here. If the patient gives a history of not being able to walk more than say 200 m without getting cramps or leg tiredness, then if they are invited to walk such a distance around the outpatient department and return, then any subtle neurological abnormalities are often considerably magnified.

Although the condition is principally one of arthritis, there is a very important soft tissue component to it and that involves the ligamentum flavum (Fig. 2.8). This is the piece of soft tissue, which conjoins the laminae at the back (the roofs of the house) and is composed to a large extent of elastic soft tissue which looks yellow, hence the name ligamentum flavum (yellow ligament). As the degenerative process continues in the posterior facet joint, the ligmentum flavum folds inwards particularly when the spine is extended, that is, with a normal lordosis (hollow back). This added soft tissue intrusion into the attic markedly increases the degree of stenosis such that it is commonly the case that patients say that they can walk but 100 or 200 m, but they can cycle all day (when you ride a bike your spine tends to be flexed, the back of the spine is stretched and any ligamentous infolding is reversed). Similarly, patients may say that they can walk much more easily upstairs when one tends to be more flexed than downstairs when one tends to have more spinal extension. Symptomatic expression is important and if the main problem is of back pain, then there is a host of non-operative treatment modalities including epidural injections, facet joint injections, ultrasound, physiotherapy, etc.

Although objective neurological dysfunction is uncommon, there is often symptomatic evidence of bladder instability. This can be increased frequency of micturition (the bladder needs to be emptied more often than normal), nocturia (having to get up in the night more often to pass urine), dribbling (the passage of a small quantity of urine after normal micturition), going on to frank incontinence, although the latter is unusual. Therefore, for the patient with spinal claudication and impending or existing neurological dysfunction, with the presence of appreciable stenosis on scanning, surgical decompression is required. In this situation, the extent of compression on the MRI scan dictates the extent of surgical decompression, which implies removal of the roofs of whatever number of houses is required to deal with the situation. At decompressive surgery, it is remarkable how stenosed the cauda equina can be, down to literally a pinhole, and yet there may be no objective neurological dysfunction, rather just symptoms therefrom. The cauda equina would normally be more than 2 cm in diameter and for it to get down to 1 mm or even less without causing paralysis is indeed remarkable.

It is not wise to remove too much of the facet joints themselves lest spinal instability is created, which in turn might raise the possibility of carrying out a concomitant spinal fusion procedure. However, the posterior facet joints can be significantly debulked just by undercutting and thus making the attic of the house larger and more triangular than trefoil. The spinous process and the posterior parts of the laminae do have to be removed, but thereafter undercutting is the method by which the spinal canal can be satisfactorily re-bored without endangering stability (Fig. 4.16).

If the scan shows one-level stenosis, then obviously only one level has to be re-bored; and if the scan shows three-level stenosis, then three levels have to be re-bored. The clinical condition of the patient in terms of symptoms and signs seldom provides sufficient information about the necessary levels of surgical decompression, and this is more reliant on the scan appearances, unlike the situation with intervertebral disc herniation, which is driven by the patient's precise symptoms and signs.

The results of surgical decompression for spinal stenosis are a bit less good than those of nerve root decompression for disc herniation, but one should be looking at an 80% success rate or thereabouts.

REFERENCES

1. Smeathers JE. Shocking news about disks. Current Orthopaedics 1994, 8: 45–48.
2. Adams MA, Dolan P. Recent advances in lumbar spinal mechanics and there recent clinical significant. Review paper. Clinical Biomechanics 1995, 10: 3–19.
3. Oner FC, van der Rijt RR, Ramos LMP, Dhert WJA, Verbout AJ. Changes in the discs space after fractures of the thoraco-lumbar spine. Journal of Bone and Joint Surgery 1998, 80-B: 833–839.
4. Battié MC, Videman T, Gibbons LE, Fisher LD, Manninen H, Gill K. Determinants of lumbar disc degeneration. A study relating lifetime exposures and magnetic resonance imaging findings in identical twins. Spine 1995, 20: 2601–2612.
5. Obukhov SK, Hankenson L, Manka M, Mawk JR. Multilevel lumbar disc herniation in 12-year-old twins. Case report. Child Nervous System 1996, 12: 169–171.
6. Kelsey JL, Gitlens PB, White III AA, Holford TR, Walker SD, O'Connor T, Ostfeld AM, Weil U, Southwick WO, Calogero JA. An epidemiologic study of lifting and twisting on the job and risk for acute prolapsed lumbar intevertebral disc. Journal of Orthopaedic Research 1984, 2: 61–66.
7. Fraser RD, Osti OL, Vernon-Roberts B. Intervertebral disc degeneration. European Spine Journal 1993, 1: 205–213.
8. Naylor A. The late results of laminectomy for lumbar disk prolapse – a review after 10–25 years. Journal of Bone and Joint Surgery 1974, 56-B: 17–29.
9. Rankine JJ, Gill PK, Hutchinson CE, Ross ERS, Williamson JB. The clinical significance of the high-intensity zone on lumbar spine magnetic resonance imaging. Spine 1999, 24(18): 1913–1920.
10. Roland M, van Tulder MW. Should radiologists change the way they report plain radiography of the spine? Viewpoint. Lancet 1998, 352: 229–230.
11. Dickson RA, Butt WP. Mini-symposium: lumbar disc disease. (I) Clinical and radiological assessment. Current Orthopaedics 1995, 9: 73–84.
12. Butt WP. Magnetic resonance imaging of the spine. Journal of Rheumatology 1994, 33: 793–797.
13. Boos N, Reider R, Schade V, Spratt KF, Semmer N, Aebi M. The diagnostic accuracy of magnetic resonance imaging, work perception, and

psychosocial factors in identifying symptomatic disc herniations. Spine 1995, 20: 2613–2625.

14. Gibson JNA, Waddell G. The surgical management of lumbar disc prolapse (protocol for a Cochrane Review). In Cochrane Library, Issue 4. 1998, Update software, Oxford.

15. Van Tulder MW, Koes BW, Bouter LM. Conservative treatment of acute and chronic non-specific low back pain. A systematic review of randomised control trials of the most common interventions. Spine 1997, 22: 2128–2156.

16. Chatterjee S, Foy PM, Findley GF. Report of a controlled clinical trial comparing automated percutaneous lumbar-discectomy and micro-discectomy in the treatment of contained lumbar disc herniation. Spine 1995, 20: 734–738.

17. Livesey JP, Sundaram S, Foster L, Peters J, Moore CA, Walker AP. Laser discectomy versus lumbar epidural steroid injection: a randomised comparative study of two treatments for sciatica. Abstract, British Orthopaedic Association, Glasgow. Journal of Bone and Joint Surgery (Br), Orthopaedic Proceedings, Suppl. 1, 2000. p 74.

18. Nachemson AL. Failed back surgery syndrome is syndrome of failed back surgeons. The Pain Clinic 1999, 11: 271–284.

19. McCulloch JA. Lumbar percutaneous disc surgery: where are we now? Current Orthopaedics 1998, 12: 77–85.

20. Waber H. Lumbar disc herniation: controlled prospective study with 10 years of observation. Spine 1983, 8: 131–140.

Spondylolisthesis

This term is derived from the two Greek words *spondyl* meaning spine and *olisthesis* meaning slippage. It most commonly occurs at the bottom of the spine – the joint between the fifth lumbar vertebra and the sacrum (the L5/S1 joint). We classify spondylolisthesis into five different types.

Types of spondylolisthesis

- Dysplastic
- Isthmic
- Traumatic
- Degenerative
- Pathological

By far the commonest is isthmic spondylolisthesis.

When spondylolisthesis occurs, the vertebra above, with the whole spine on top of it, slips forward on the one below. Having vertebrae slipping around sounds a dreadful situation but, with few exceptions, the condition is much more benign than one would think.

DYSPLASTIC SPONDYLOLISTHESIS

Dysplastic means abnormal formation and the dysplasia in question concerns the posterior facet joint at the back of the spine, which quite simply has not formed properly (embryological failure for whatever reason). You will recall from the earlier biomechanics section that the posterior facet joint aids stability and if it has not formed properly then it may be incompetent in its ability to prevent movement. While the dysplasia is *congenital* (present at or before birth), slippage may never occur and thus, the dysplasia or even *aplasia* (no facet joint formed at all) may never be recognised.

Conversely, because the defect is present at or before birth, then the degree of slippage can be considerable, sometimes so much so that the fifth lumbar vertebra actually rolls round a full 90° to lie in front of the sacrum – where the rectum would normally be (Figs 5.1a–c). Not surprisingly, it was

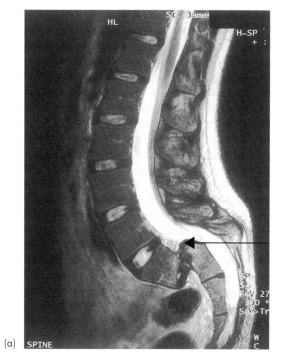

(a)

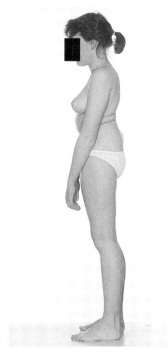

(b)

Fig. 5.1   (continued).

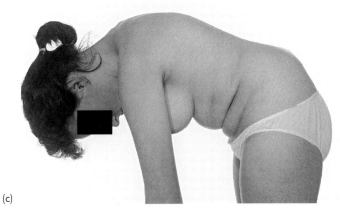

(c)

Fig. 5.1 (a) Sagittal lumbar MRI scan showing that the bottom lumbar vertebra (L5), which should be sitting on top of the sacrum (arrow) has in fact rolled to sit on the front of S1. This is the most severe degree of dysplastic spondylolisthesis referred to as spondyloptosis. Apart from a skin crease in the (b) erect position and a moderate angular deformity on (c) bending forward, this young lady was entirely symptom free with no pain. These pictures were taken, when she was 17 and she is now in her early 30s with no clinical problems.

obstetricians, a couple of 100 years ago, who first recognised the significance of dysplastic spondylolisthesis simply because the baby's head would not go through the birth passages and, in an effort to save the mother's life, the unborn child often had to be sacrificed.

ISTHMIC SPONDYLOLISTHESIS

The *isthmus* is that part of the posterior vertebral arch (the roof of the house) that lies between the superior and inferior facet. A defect in the isthmus can allow the vertebral body and posterior arch behind the isthmus to separate (the body of the house and the roof part company). As the electrical clockwork lies between the house and the roof, the space for it is actually enlarged in isthmic spondylolisthesis, and so neurological consequences are exceptional.

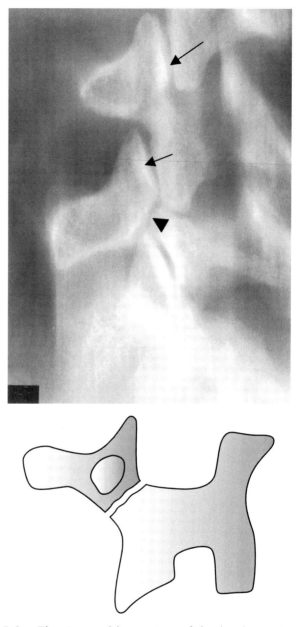

Fig. 5.2   This is an oblique view of the lumbar spine, which shows the posterior facet joints (arrows) and the bone between them. This oblique lumbar spine appearance has been likened to a scotty dog. If the scotty dog has a collar (arrowhead) this is a spondylolysis or crack fracture and this oblique view is particularly useful in identifying such a lesion.

The cause of isthmic spondylolisthesis is a stress or fatigue fracture across the isthmus, which is very much more common than is generally appreciated (Fig. 5.2). Even using the fairly crude routine frontal and lateral X-rays (which are by no means the best angles to spot a stress fracture) the prevalence rate is estimated to be of the order of 3% of 3-year olds rising to 8–10% of teenagers and young adults and 50% of Eskimos for whatever reason! There is a much higher incidence in children/adolescents, who arch their back frequently and appreciably, such as ballet dancers, gymnasts (Fig. 5.3), trampolinists and fast bowlers (as many as 20% or more), and so it is thought

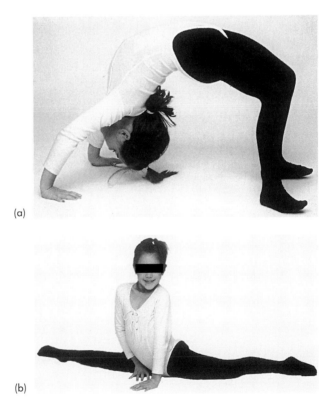

(a)

(b)

Fig. 5.3   As soon as this little 10-year-old girl came into clinic complaining of low-back pain an early question had to be "are you a (a) gymnast or a (b) ballet dancer?" Not surprisingly the answer was yes to both. X-rays showed bilateral lyses but no slippage. It is this repetitive arching and twisting of the back that produces lyses in the first place and then subsequently on occasion renders them symptomatic.

that repetitive arching and possibly twisting of the back during the formative years eventually can lead to a stress fracture and can produce symptoms from established lyses.

It would appear that in many individuals the fracture goes on to heal and these people leave the prevalence pool, while new cases enter but, in any event, spondylolyses do not heal (unless we help) after the attainment of skeletal maturity, which for the spine may not be until the early 20s. These stress fractures then remain for life. As they are so prevalent, they are very often seen on low-back X-rays taken in individuals who, for example, have sustained a typical low-back soft tissue strain. Unfortunately for no very good reason, since they belong to the one in 10 at least who have a stress fracture, all their problems may be incorrectly attributed to that (more of this later). Rather like the posterior facet joint incompetence in dysplastic spondylolisthesis, the stress fracture can lead to slippage and, therefore, frank spondylolisthesis. It can, however, also be painful in its own right. Spinal surgeons not uncommonly see teenagers (young adults), who are high sporting achievers who repetitively break down when they play their sport at the highest level. Plain films show no evidence of spondylolisthesis but oblique films taken at 45°, which better lines up the isthmus or computerised tomographic (CT) scanning confirms the presence of the stress fracture.

Stress fractures can be present on one side (i.e. right or left isthmus) or bilaterally and of course only if the lyses are present bilaterally can slippage and spondylolisthesis occur. Clearly, the prognosis is going to be a lot better if the defect is present only on one side (Fig. 5.4). When the lyses are bilateral and spondylolisthesis occurs this probably happens in about a quarter of individuals who have lyses and so possibly as many as 3–5% of the population do have a spondylolisthesis albeit generally of a minor degree.

When there is such a seemingly obvious mechanical low-back problem with such a high prevalence rate in the community at large one should be seeing these patients with recalcitrant low-back pain in their droves but that is not so to the point where one has to question whether, at least in the adult with low-back pain, the presence of a spondylolisthesis is really clinically relevant at all. It is different in the more active teenager,

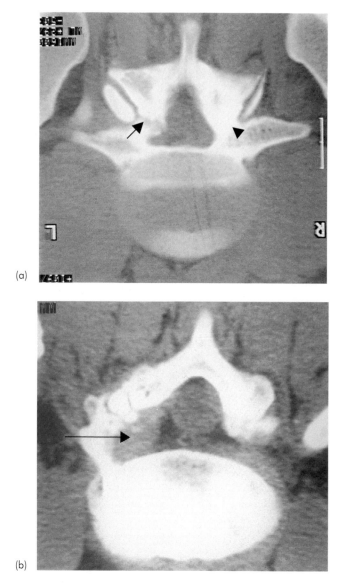

(a)

(b)

Fig. 5.4 (a) Axial CT scan shows that there is only a lysis on the left side (arrow) but there is a lot of protective thickening of the same part of the vertebra on the right side as the secondary mechanism (arrowhead). (b) Axial MRI shows that the lysis is surrounded by a considerable mass of repair debris just where the local exiting nerve root would be (arrow). Sciatica is, therefore, occasionally produced but it is exceptional for this to be accompanied by muscle weakness or sensory reduction.

where changes of shape with growth compound the situation and we certainly recognise spondylolisthesis as being a notable cause of back pain in this age group, but with the attainment of maturity the condition stabilises. Neither new spondylolyses occur after the attainment of maturity (i.e. those spotted in, say, the 20s have been present for probably a decade) nor do any degrees of spondylolisthesis progress beyond maturity, rather spondylolistheses *stabilise,* when the individual is fully grown. Indeed, radiological studies have clearly shown that X-ray evidence of spondylolisthesis in the adult is not a risk factor for back pain (see Chapter 8; Ref. 18).

Therefore, once the owner stops growing the presence of the bilateral defects in the isthmus are nothing more than an additional posterior facet joint. When we operate on patients with spondylolisthesis, this fragment between the *new joint* and the proper facet joint below, the so-called *rattle fragment*, is very loose but the rest of the intervertebral joint is intact. The muscles and ligaments at the back of the spine in the lower-lumbar region are well known to skip a few levels (i.e. they are not attached at every single level) and, therefore, it is not easy to see why the presence of bilateral spondylolyses or a spondylolisthesis should necessarily be *unstable* on any anatomical or biomechanical considerations.

Prior to MRI scanning, particularly in the days of myelography and then CT scanning, it was felt that *instability* was more obvious in spondylolisthesis patients because of the apparent higher prevalence rate of intervertebral disc protrusions at the level of the slip, and indeed at the level above it. However, with the advent of MRI scanning, when it looks as though everybody has a disc problem, many patients with quite obvious spondylolisthesis have entirely pristine discs with no evidence of degeneration. Such an MRI finding is not at all uncommon and then begs the question as to whether spondylolisthesis is at all unstable or if it is whether *instability* is a risk factor for disc degeneration. It is clearly not in the rest of the population and so why should it be in the spondylolisthesis patient? Or is it that the same bad genes that produce pre-mature disc degeneration also produce spondylolyses/spondylolisthesis? There is a much higher incidence in family members indicating a strong genetic trend. There certainly are no data available to indicate that spondylolyses/spondylolisthesis in the adult indicate a state of vulnerability to either an increased frequency, severity or duration of low-back pain and, with a condition as prevalent as it is, one would expect such data to have been presented long ago. Furthermore, as these basic prevalence rates of 3% of 3-year olds and 8–10% of teenagers with a spondylolysis are based upon crude frontal and lateral films and not the oblique views or CT scanning that we commonly use to investigate our low-back patients, the prevalence rates can probably be confidently doubled to the point, where it is certainly not *statistically abnormal* to have an isthmic defect in the first place. It certainly seems very simplistic to believe that one low-back strain has initiated in a 50-year old at work a saga of low-back problems sufficient to stop him working for the next 15 years, just because an X-ray shows spondylolyses of 40 years duration. Epidemiological studies would not support such a proposition. Surely 50% of Eskimos are not disabled by back pain!

Treatment of dysplastic and isthmic spondylolisthesis

As it is repetitive stressing of the low back, which produces symptoms then for children/adolescents with spondylolisthesis a reduction in physical activity, such as sports, generally leads to relief of symptoms but occasionally, because of severe relacitrant low-back pain or increasing slip (much more common with dysplastic than isthmic), we prescribe a spinal fusion operation which, if the spondylolisthesis was at the L5/S1 level, would fuse together the lowest lumbar vertebra to the sacrum (the bones on each side) so that a joint would no longer exist (Figs 5.5a–d and 5.5e, f). The notion behind this is that movement produces symptoms and, therefore, the abolition of movement will abolish symptoms and that happy situation does occur in probably 90% of cases. The fusion is carried out by roughening up the two bones and putting on the roughened surfaces some pieces of bone taken from the inside of the pelvis. This harvested bone is superfluous to requirements (like 90% of your liver) and leaves no disability in the young. This bone graft then unites to the fifth lumbar and first sacral vertebrae and joins them like a fracture heals. Sound bony union is,

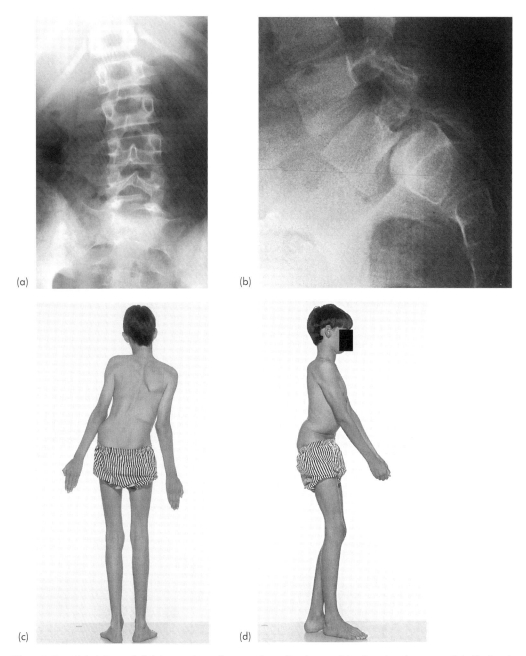

Fig. 5.5 (a) AP and (b) lateral radiographs of a boy with dysplastic spondylolisthesis of about 50%. Note the list to the side on the frontal film due to muscle spasm. (c) Back and (d) side view of this boy of 14. This deformity is entirely due to muscle spasm secondary to the pain of the spondylolisthesis. This is called the "adolescent crisis".

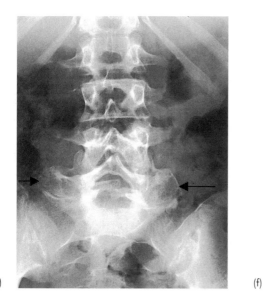
(e)

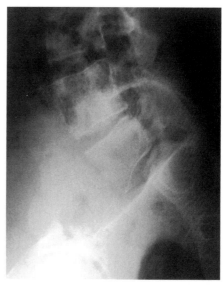
(f)

Fig. 5.5   (e) AP and (f) lateral views 2 years after surgery showing a solid fusion (arrows) and a straight spine. There was no visible deformity at follow-up and the young man had actually grown 5 in.

therefore, not reached for several months until the *fracture* has consolidated.

The adult presenting with low-back pain in association with spondylolyses or spondylolisthesis may also fail standard non-operative therapy (e.g. rest, spinal support, painkillers, physiotherapy, epidural injections, etc.) and be dealt with in a similar fashion surgically by way of a spinal fusion, although the results are much less satisfactory, probably no higher than 60% success. The older individual with the bigger skeleton can generally receive internal metalwork, which holds the bones together internally until the bone graft unites and this saves the patient from having to wear a post-operative spinal support, although there is no evidence that a one level lumbar spine fusion requires either internal (metalwork) or external (brace) support. Moreover, pedicular screws can stray from their desired location and traumatise the local nerve root. Neurological complications can, therefore, occur with metalwork, which would not occur with a straightforward non-instrumented fusion. Surely the patient should be informed about this sort of matter. Surgery is not an inconsiderable undertaking in that for anyone with anything more than a very sedentary job up to a year off work is probably required to return to reasonable fitness.

In the adult, the spondylolysis has undergone frustrated attempts at bony union and, therefore, the gap seen as the lysis on the X-ray is not fresh air but rather is gristle, which is not ossified but may contain some calcium. It is in reality a heaping up of partly calcified gristle and as the nerve root runs right underneath the lysis then if there is a big enough heaping up of tissue the local nerve root can be irritated (Fig. 5.4). Therefore, in the adult, low-back pain can be accompanied by sciatica and thus the nerve root in question might need to be cleared by removal of the gristle at the same time as the fusion procedure is carried out. True nerve root compression rather than just irritation is, however, exceptional.

TRAUMATIC SPONDYLOLISTHESIS

If someone has a fracture–dislocation of the spine and an X-ray taken from the side shows loss of alignment (i.e. one vertebra is in front or behind the one next to it) then this can be referred to as traumatic spondylolisthesis (Fig. 2.7). However, this is unnecessary classification ITIS. Rather this so-called *traumatic spondylolisthesis* should belong to the classification of spinal fracture–dislocations (see later) and not of spondylolisthesis.

DEGENERATIVE SPONDYLOLISTHESIS

In primary degenerative osteoarthritis, with the pathology that we have seen closely resembling degenerative disc disease, the posterior facet joints can be attacked and, therefore, wear. This can lead to incompetence much as the dysplastic form of spondylolisthesis does in children. The typical patient is the middle aged/early elderly female (females are very susceptible to primary generalised osteoarthritis because it is genetic like disc disease), the L4/5 level is much the most common, and because slippage occurs without the presence of an isthmic

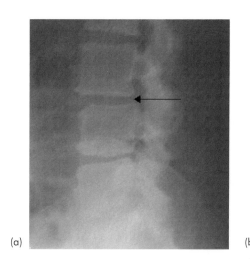
(a)

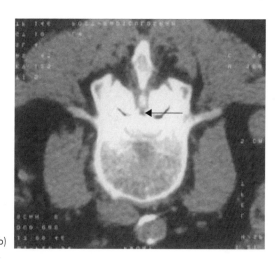
(b)

Fig. 5.6 *Degenerative spondylolisthesis.* (a) Lateral X-ray showing only a slight degree of forward slippage between the third and fourth lumbar vertebrae, perhaps only 2 mm (arrow). (b) Axial CT scan showing about 1 mm of space for the nerves of the cauda equina (arrow). Surprisingly, apart from some aches in the calves after walking a quarter of a mile, there were no other symptoms.

defect the cauda equina can become progressively compressed. The body of the house and the roof do not part company, rather one entire house slips on the next so that the clockwork in the attic is sheared (guillotined or scissored). Indeed because of the new bone formation in association with the arthritic process responsible for the slippage, not more than a millimetre or two of spondylolisthesis can result in a complete block to the passage of the cauda equina (Fig. 5.6). Fortunately, neurological tissue is forgiving when the compressive process takes decades to occur. It is, therefore, unusual to have frank neurological signs and the diagnosis is made by way of low-back pain in association with the typical features of spinal canal stenosis – namely cramps and tiredness in the legs, usually exercise related and frequently symptoms of bladder instability (increased frequency, stress incontinence, dribbling, etc.).

After MRI confirmation of the diagnosis, treatment is by surgical decompression of whatever bone is pressing on the cauda equina followed by instrumented fusion of that particular joint because the facets themselves are the cause of the stenosis and their complete removal is essential for adequate decompression.

PATHOLOGICAL SPONDYLOLISTHESIS

Some *pathological* conditions, such as rheumatoid arthritis, Paget's disease (Fig. 5.7) and secondary cancer, can lead to erosion of bone or joint resulting in slippage between two adjacent vertebrae. Neurological dysfunction is common.

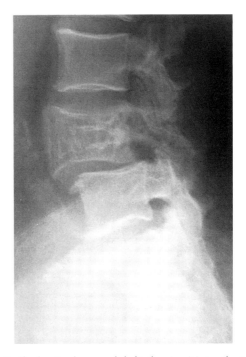

Fig. 5.7 *Pathological spondylolisthesis.* Note that the fourth lumbar vertebra has moved appreciably forward on the fifth, is a bit bigger than the vertebrae above and below, and has the typical course and irregular appearance of a Pagetic vertebra.

CHAPTER 6

Spinal Fractures and Dislocations

While soft tissue musculo-ligamentous strains and contusions occur with fairly low violence once the energy considerations rise appreciably then the spinal column is open to significant structural failure. Bones can be broken (fractures), joints can be torn apart (dislocations) and an injury can have a bit of both (fracture–dislocation).

The prevalence of these injuries is rising all the while, mostly in association with steadily increasing traffic density, and the incidence of paralysis is approaching one hundred per million population per year. Neck (cervical) injuries are the commonest, being more than twice as frequent as thoracic injuries with lumbar injuries in between. This is because the neck and lower back have much bigger ranges of motion, while the intervening thoracic intervertebral joints allow much less motion and are further splinted by the attached chest wall (ribs and breast bone). It, therefore, takes bigger energies to fracture or dislocate the thoracic spine and, moreover, there is much less space in the thoracic spine for the spinal cord compared to the cervical and lumbar regions. Not surprisingly, paralysis in association with thoracic spinal injuries is twice as common as with lumbar injuries (43% versus 21%) (Table 6.1).

While the paralysis rate seems very high, the majority fortunately recover and it is important to differentiate patients with complete paralysis on admission from those with partial paralysis since the latter have a very much better prognosis for neurological recovery. It is, therefore, essential to assess these patients neurologically accurately and as early as possible as a baseline so that this can be compared with subsequent assessments. This is not the very detailed neurological examination that might be required to localise a tumour to a particular part of the brain or spinal cord, and indeed it would not be to the

Table 6.1 Five-year figures of major spinal trauma from a level 1 Canadian Trauma Centre.

	Cervical	Thoracic	Lumbar	Total
Fractures–dislocations				
No neurological injury	436 (43%)	205 (20%)	382 (37%)	1023 (100%)
With neurological injury	171 (36%)	206 (43%)	103 (21%)	480 (100%)
Total spinal injuries	606 (40%)	410 (27%)	484 (33%)	1503 (100%)

patient's advantage to have unnecessary treatment time wasted by too fussy an assessment. Rather, it is a summary evaluation of muscle (motor) power, touch (sensation) and reflexes (in the limbs and anus).

As we go down the spinal cord from the top of the neck to the sacrum, major nerve branches come out at each level and we know where these nerves go to, so that when we test certain parts of the arms and legs we know which spinal level supplies this area. For instance, if there is a neck injury above the fourth cervical level, then the nerves that supply all the muscles of respiration are damaged in which case the patients cannot breathe for themselves. Clearly in this situation, death is a likely outcome but if a medical team can get to the scene of the accident sufficiently quickly, then the patient can be breathed for and they can in fact survive, as did the film actor Christopher Reeve. As the first spinal level to move the shoulder is the C5 level then if someone is resuscitated and breathed for and survives then no limb movements are possible. As we go down the arms successive spinal levels supply successively distal (further down the limb) muscle groups. C5 moves the shoulder, C6 and 7 move the elbow, and C7/8 and the first thoracic level (T1) move the wrist, hand and fingers.

Going down to the lower extremities the same pattern prevails with spinal levels staggered one more distally as we go down the joints. L2, 3, 4, 5 move the hips, and L3, 4, 5, S1 move the knees, L4, 5, S1, 2 move the ankles and toes, and then S3, 4, 5 supply the muscle of the anus and the skin surrounding it.

Between the neck and lumbar spine, the thoracic spinal cord and its segmental branches supply stripes of skin from the bottom of neck to groin as well as the muscles between the ribs (intercostal muscles) that do some breathing and the muscles of the front of the abdomen, which contain the abdominal organs as well as flexing the spine.

We then can localise the level of cord damage and we refer to the level as the last one which functions. Thus, if in a neck injury the person can move their shoulders but nothing more distally (i.e. paralysis from elbow downwards), then this is a C5 level.

As it is not easy to localise loss of thoraco-abdominal muscle function, we rely in the trunk more on the assessment of sensation. Thus, if the person can feel their trunk down to the umbilicus but not lower, then this is the tenth thoracic level and that level of paralysis would be referred to as T10.

We just saw that hip movements were carried out by four consecutive levels (L2, 3, 4, 5). L2 and 3 supply the muscles that flex the hip, and L4 and 5 the muscles that extend the hip. If, therefore, the patient can flex their hip only but cannot extend the hip or move the knee, ankle or toes, this implies that there is no function below L3. In addition to assessing motor function in this fashion we also measure the power of it. The need to do so became overwhelmingly obvious following the World Wars during which there were so many nerve injuries sustained. A gold standard was necessary to determine how bad the degree of nerve damage was to begin with and just as importantly how well the patient was doing after treatment. The Medical Research Council (MRC) in the UK were asked to look into this matter and produced six grades of muscle power (Table 6.2). They thought that it ought to be possible for anybody evaluating such patients to assign the appropriate grade and thus be able to easily discriminate between two consecutive levels of power. Clearly no power and normal power (grades 0 and 5, respectively) are easy to determine. Similarly, just a flicker of power (grade 1) would also be easy to assign as well as almost full power (grade 4). To differentiate between grades 2 and 3 muscle function, they incorporated the notion of muscle contraction against (grade 3) and not against (grade 2) gravity. For instance, if the patient is lying supine (on their back) and can just flex their hip (obviously against gravity) but not sufficient for a grade 4 rating, then this represents grade 3 function; if they cannot flex their hip lying supine but can do so on their side (when gravity is eliminated), this is grade 2 function.

Table 6.2 MRC grading of muscle power.

0	No power
1	Flicker
2	Movement but *not* against gravity
3	Movement against gravity
4	Movement against gravity plus some resistance
5	Normal power

There is no comparable grading system for testing touch and, therefore, this is measured descriptively, for example, normal, absent and reduced.

The nerve which leaves the spine at each level contains both motor and sensory fibres as well as some funny ones called autonomic nerves which make the bowels work, keep the heart going and make one blush or have goose pimples. Just as we know the level of paralysis from the last working muscle so we can determine the level of sensory damage. We have already said that the sensory nerves supply certain stripes or patches called dermatomes and in someone with complete cord damage, say at C5, then sensation would be preserved in the C5 dermatome over the shoulder and upper part of the arm but there would be no sensation below.

Fortunately, and importantly, the majority of paralyses are incomplete, only affecting a part of the spinal cord. Motor nerves tend to run down the front of the cord, while sensory nerves run down the back. Therefore, if only the front part of the cord is involved (*anterior cord syndrome*) there can be reduced motor power in the presence of normal sensation and vice versa for damage to the back of the cord. This *posterior cord syndrome* is, however, very rarely encountered clinically. Then the nerve supply to the arms tends to come from the middle of the cord in the neck and that to the legs comes from the outer part of the cord. Therefore, with a *central cord syndrome* the arms may not work but the legs may do. Then finally, you can have an injury to one side of the cord and because different types of nerves run down different parts of the cord a side lesion gives rise to paralysis on the same side and reduction of sensation on the other side. This is called the *Brown-Séquard syndrome*. Therefore, a brief 15-min assessment, if time allows, will demonstrate the presence of complete or incomplete paralysis, if complete at what level, and if incomplete to what degree, and if differences between motor and sensory function are detected whether the lesion is in the front, the back, the middle or the side of the cord. This is of important prognostic significance. Obviously, complete cord lesions have a less good prognosis whereas central cord lesions and Brown-Séquard syndromes are more forgiving.

Finally, the neurological assessment of the spinal injury patient is not complete without adequate assessment of the *perineum* (the peri-anal and the genital areas). For a few inches around the anus the skin is supplied by the S3, 4 and 5 roots and with a pin (not the much sharper needle which can draw blood and cause much more discomfort) this area can be quickly tested as regards sensation (Fig. 6.1). Importantly, the skin immediately around the anus is supplied by the S5 dermatome and if this is stimulated by a pin then normally the anus will reflexly contract (the *anal wink*).

Then a rectal examination should be carried out to determine the status of the anal sphincter. With a normal per rectum (PR) examination, the anal sphincter can be found to be contractile with some initial difficulty in finger insertion and then if the patient is asked to contract the anal sphincter and tug down on the finger, further information about the anal sphincter can be gleaned. A good tug indicates normal function whereas no tug or a weak tug indicates a precarious situation. Then with the finger still in the rectum, the penis or clitoris can be gently squeezed, or the catheter tugged, and if this leads to contraction of the anal sphincter (i.e. a tug round the finger)

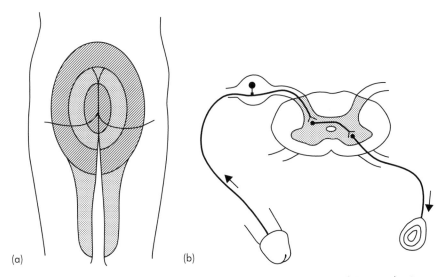

(a)   (b)

Fig. 6.1 *Assessing the perineum.* (a) The sacral nerves 3, 4 and 5 supply rings of skin around the anus. (b) Squeezing the penis should normally produce contraction of the anal sphincter. These two simple tests, combined with a rectal examination, take less than a minute to perform, but constitute an essential template against which further assessments can be measured. From Dickson RA (1990). Spinal Surgery – Science and Practice. Butterworths, London & Boston.

then this is a normal reflex (the bulbo-cavernosus). Doing this test followed by no tug round the finger would indicate absence of this reflex.

This completes the initial neurological assessment of the patient and it takes in reality no more than 15 min to accomplish and, with experience, can be accomplished much more quickly should other matters (such as a serious head, chest or abdominal injury) prevail at the same time. Thus, this initial assessment followed by further assessments according to need can help to establish fairly firmly a reasonably accurate prognosis.

After a significant spinal cord injury there can follow a phase of what is described as *spinal shock*. This is a temporary loss of electrical nerve transmission down the spinal cord because it is concussed. This is a shock to the cord sufficient to temporarily knock it out of action but not sufficient to contuse or damage the cord in the majority of cases.

This state of spinal cord shock or concussion can last for a matter of a few seconds, through a few minutes, or hours, to even a day or, uncommonly, more than that. During this period of electrical failure, everything is knocked out like a power cut and there is simply no neurological response. There is no movement and no sensation and no reflexes. It is important to appreciate that reflexes, by the very nature of the word, are not under voluntary control and are mediated by the spinal cord itself. As spinal shock wears off, these reflexes return indicating that the spinal cord is recovering electrically. The return of reflexes should be accompanied by a return of sensation and motor power but if that does not happen by the time the reflexes return then the prognosis is very bad with virtually no chance of any muscle power or sensation recovering and, therefore, permanent paralysis. The longer the period of spinal shock persists the less likely it is that full recovery will occur. This reinforces the important point that neurological assessment must be carried out adequately and early enough and repeated so that the natural history and prognosis of the spinal cord insult can be properly appreciated.

All this concern about the function of the spinal cord is because the central nervous system (brain and spinal cord) has no power of recovery after frank nerve damage. It can recover after concussion or shock but not direct nerve damage. The muscles and ligaments along with the bones of the spine, which are the spine's shock absorbers, do have the ability to heal and restore mechanical spinal column integrity but unfortunately the spinal cord does not have that innate ability. However, once the branches have been given off from the spinal cord at each level (this is referred to as the peripheral, rather than the central, nervous system), these peripheral nerves do have the ability to regenerate when damaged and, accordingly, recovery from peripheral nerve damage is very much on the cards, although the more proximal the damage the further the regenerating nerves have to travel and, therefore, the worse the prognosis.

Knowing the nature and extent of damage to the spinal column is useful in determining the likelihood of both neurological and mechanical disability. Over the years a number of classifications of the extent of spinal column damage have been proposed; early on Prof. Holdsworth in Sheffield suggested a simple two-part (front–back) classification based upon his not inconsiderable experience with spinal injuries in coal miners (who were working on all fours or in a stooped position when coal above fell on them with considerable force, paralysing many). Figure 6.2 shows his anterior and posterior two-column concept which is basically that the house is the front (anterior) column and the roof is the back (posterior) column. This theory has a lot to commend it. The house is the compression part of the spinal column represented by the vertebral bodies and discs with the anterior longitudinal ligament in front of it and the posterior longitudinal ligament behind it whereas the roof represents the tension members with the pedicles, laminae, spinous processes and transverse processes, with their connecting muscles and ligaments. Remember that to resist tension or stretching it is tensile strength that is required and this can be achieved by ropes or cables of fairly small diameter whereas compression requires much bigger dimension pillars or columns.

The antithesis of the simple Holdsworth two-column theory is the modern Association of Osteosynthesis (AO) Swiss classification, which has evolved over the past three decades from the ever-burgeoning worldwide experience of internal fixation of fractures using metalwork developed by the Swiss internal fixation AO group. AO classifications have letters (A, B, C) and numbers (1, 2, 3) and various permutations and combinations

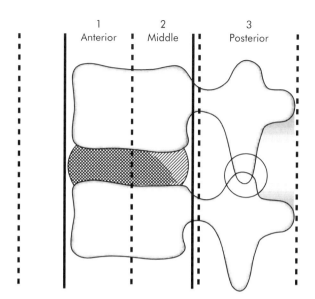

Fig. 6.2 *The spinal columns*. Sir Frank Holdsworth described just two columns – front and back – while Denis suggested three columns – anterior, middle and posterior. Holdsworth's anterior column comprises both the anterior and middle columns of Denis. From Dickson RA (1990). Spinal Surgery – Science and Practice. Butterworths, London & Boston.

of letters and numbers describe the full gamut of injuries that can happen.

Happily, in between, there is a much less busy classification proposed by Francis Denis of Minneapolis who extended Holdsworth's two-column theory to a three-column one. He divided Holdsworth's anterior compression column into two and so column 1 is the front half of the bodies and discs, column 2 is the back half of the bodies and discs, and column 3 is Holdsworth's posterior column (Fig. 6.2).

Denis' classification sought to help in determining the extent and stability of spinal injuries and, therefore, some rationale underpinning their management. Indeed in the simplest terms, Denis' three-column concept states that the more columns that are disrupted, the more unstable the injury is and the more need for providing stability by way of treatment. He proposes four fundamental injury types based upon damage to one or more columns. For instance, simple compression of the anterior half of a vertebra (anterior column) is a straightforward

Table 6.3 Spinal column involvement in the different injury types (Denis).

Type of fracture	Anterior	Middle	Posterior
Compression	Compression	None	None or distraction (severe)
Burst	Compression	Compression	None
Seat-belt type	None or compression	Distraction	Distraction
Fracture–dislocation	Compression rotation shear	Distraction rotation shear	Distraction rotation shear

vertebral wedge compression fracture, which is the simplest type of bony injury to understand. The front of the vertebral body is squashed down, usually not more than by a quarter to a half and the rest of the spine is left intact (Table 6.3).

With a simple wedge compression fracture the spine is still very stable because the front of the vertebra is squashed into itself rather like a great white shark's teeth being clamped together; once the force that caused the injury has finished then the two sets of interlocking teeth prevent movement in any direction and the injury is *stable*. Therefore, after the initial phase of pain locally, which may require temporary hospitalisation and a week or two of external orthotic support, patients are relatively symptom-free and can be mobilised forthwith. This injury is two a penny in jockeys who are back in the saddle, whether advisedly or not, within a few weeks. If the wedge compression injury only involves one vertebra then the resultant degree of kyphosis is of no consequence either mechanically or as regards deformity. Not infrequently, however, the anterior vertebral wedging can extend over a number of vertebrae and, thus, while the biomechanical consequences remain the same, the deformity may be appreciable. As the middle of the spinal column is at the lower thoracic region, then this is where vertebral compression fracturing tends to occur. It is also precisely the same area as a developmental type of vertebral wedging occurs referred to as *thoracic hyperkyphosis* or *Scheuermann's disease*. Expert witnesses may well be asked to address the question as to whether the injury produced two or three level anterior vertebral traumatic compression wedging or whether the problem is of long-standing Scheuermann's disease. Obviously pre-injury films will be important, if such exist, but there are features of fresh injury which help to differentiate the two – buckling of the anterior vertebral sur-face (Fig. 6.3) along with soft tissue swelling representing fresh haemorrhage. End-plate irregularities and antero-posterior elongation of the vertebral bodies are the characteristics of Scheuermann's disease. After a short symptomatic period the prognosis of wedge compression injuries is excellent and cer-tainly no local pain would be expected in the long term. The great majority of such individuals ought to be able to return within a matter of a few months to their pre-injury occupa-tion. As it is the vertebra that is squashed down and there is no joint damage, then there is no risk of future degenerative arthritis.

The next fundamental type of Denis' bony injuries is referred to as the *burst fracture*. This is much the same injury mechanism as the anterior wedge compression injury but the forces are a

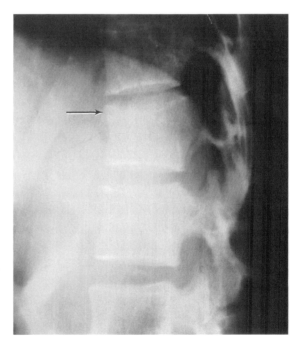

Fig. 6.3 *A wedge compression fracture.* The front surface of the vertebra is squashed a bit producing obvious buckling (arrow). Note that the front height of the vertebral body is obvi-ously less than those above and below. This buckling will remodel and, therefore, its presence indicates a fresh injury.

bit bigger and a bit more vertically orientated and so one of the key features of a burst fracture is reduction in height of the back of the vertebral body (Denis' second column) as well as the front. If you can imagine the vertebral body being rather like a meringue and if you hit downwards upon it with your fist, cream will fly in all directions. The vertebrae are, however, surrounded by strong ligaments, which are stretched during this process and then contract to bring the cream back inwards again. Behind the vertebral bodies, in the attic of the house, is the spinal cord. The meringue model of course has cream in the middle but in the biological situation the cream is represented by bone fragments which pass backwards and can impart considerable damage to the spinal cord. Then the ligaments surrounding the vertebral bodies and discs recoil the cream so that the X-rays and scans in the casualty department may reflect only a fraction of what happened at the instantaneous moment of injury (Figs 6.4a, b and 6.4 c–e). An important point here is that, looking at the spine from the side, the front of the bodies are

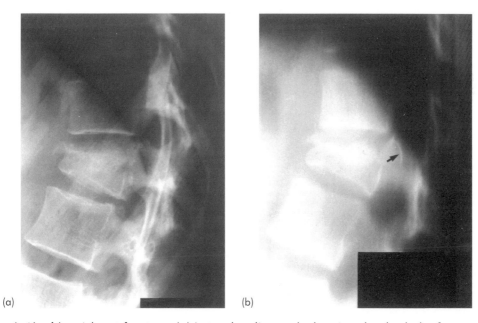

(a)   (b)

Fig. 6.4(a, b) *A burst fracture.* (a) Lateral radiograph showing that both the front and back height of the vertebral body are reduced. Look at the vertebrae above and below to see what the normal sort of height should be. (b) Lateral tomogram (a radiographic slice through the middle of the vertebra) showing that there is a large fragment of bone pushed backwards where the spinal cord would be (arrow).

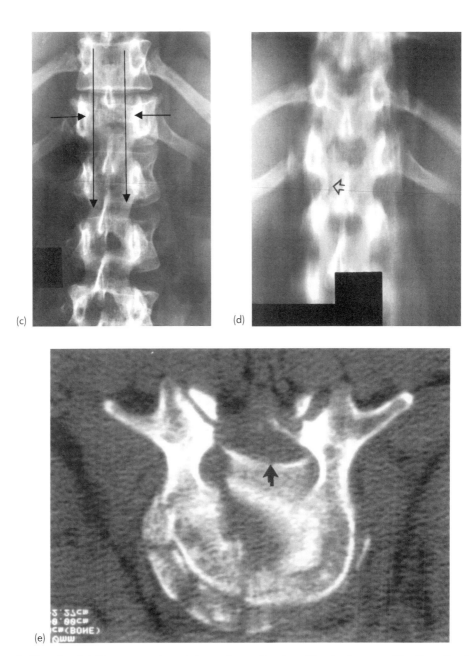

Fig. 6.4(c–e)   (c) The second vertebrae from the top (the last one with ribs attached) has its pedicles a bit widened (arrows) (with a burst fracture everything is squashed outwards). (d) AP tomogram through the posterior column showing the obligatory lamina crack (arrow) typical of a burst fracture. (e) Axial CT scan showing the retropulsed fragment (arrow) in the spinal canal.

squashed more than the back of the bodies (Denis' columns 1 and 2) whereas the back of the spine (Denis' column 3) is not squashed but there always is a crack in the lamina at the back of the burst vertebra and so it looks to all intents and purposes as though this might be a three-column (anterior, middle and posterior) rather than a two-column (anterior and middle) injury. Remember that the posterior column resists tension because of the many attached muscles and ligaments and a crack in a lamina at the back does not reduce the tensile strength of the posterior column. In simple terms, therefore, while the vertebral body might be squashed down, the back is essentially intact and these injuries are very much more stable than is often considered.

The third type of injury according to Denis occurs when the spinal column flexes over the seat-belt so that the fulcrum of the injury is actually in front of the spine. This is nicely exemplified by the gymnast doing a routine on the parallel bars. Part of the routine involves the tummy going towards, making contact with the bar, and then flexing over it. The bar represents the fulcrum and everything behind it must, therefore, be stretched (under tension). This is rather like a book being opened with the parallel bar being a bit in front of the spine of the book (Fig. 6.5). Now the whole spine is under tension and the spine does indeed open like a book. This can occur through the vertebral body itself or can occur through the posterior facet joints and the disc end-plate junction (i.e. through soft tissue). This injury was first described by Dr Chance, a radiologist. It was subsequently called a seat-belt injury in the days, when seat-belts had a lap construct only rather than a lap and diagonal which prevents this type of injury, but now it is usually called a Chance's fracture. Therefore, while this may appear to be a three-column injury it is in fact generally stable because after the moment of injury when the book opens, the book then closes and the asperities of the fracture surfaces (great white shark's or crocodile's teeth) lock together to reconfer stability. The soft tissue disc end-plate junction and facet Chance injury is, of course, much less stable.

The fourth and final type of injury is the fracture–dislocation, where all three columns are disrupted and there can be significant movement (translation) of the spine above with reference to the spine below (Fig. 6.6). This exerts a shearing force on the

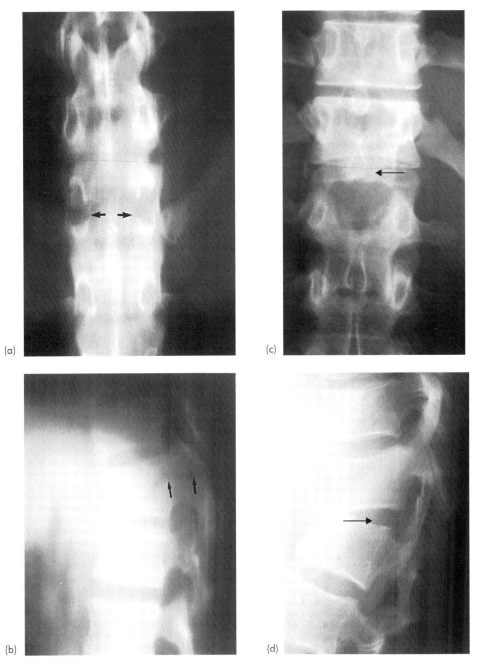

Fig. 6.5 *The seat-belt or "Chance" fracture.* Here the fulcrum is in front of the spine which is the binding of the book. The book opens up progressively more backwards. (a, b) Chance fracture through the vertebral body (arrows). (c, d) In another case the injury has occurred through the end-plate disc junction and facet joint (arrows).

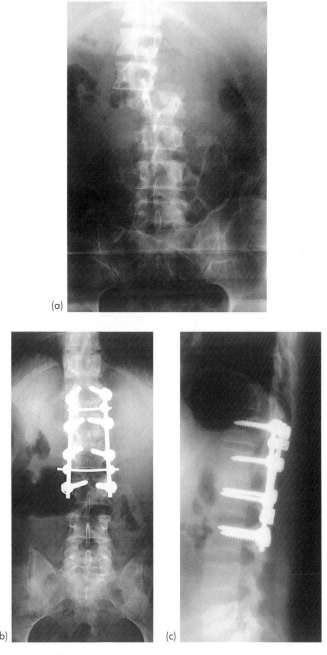

Fig. 6.6 *A very serious fracture–dislocation of the upper lumbar spine.* (a) Considerable shift of the upper lumbar spine to the side. (b) AP and (c) lateral radiographs after open reduction and internal fixation. Extraordinarily despite an initial complete paralysis, this man eventually managed to walk out of hospital and fathered a child the next year!

contained spinal cord and, not surprisingly, with all three columns disrupted with shearing, there is a high incidence of spinal cord damage. The majority of these injuries occur at the junction of the thoracic and lumbar spines, because of their relatively different bending and stiffness characteristics, and a variety of different neurological problems can result. We have already seen that the spinal cord tends to end at the bottom of L1 and, therefore, if the injury occurs much above this level it can compromise the spinal cord. If the injury occurs lower, or indeed the spinal cord ends, for whatever reason, higher, then the resultant neurological injury affects more the cauda equina than the cord with, therefore, sparing of certain nerve roots.

In injuries of the spinal column you will have doubtless heard about two different neurological scenarios – *upper motor neurone signs and lower motor neurone signs*. If the central nervous system (brain and spinal cord) are injured then we have what are called upper motor neurone signs. This means that the reflexes are greatly exaggerated, movements are difficult to elicit because of stiffness (hypertonic) and scratching the feet (the plantar responses) makes the big toes turn upwards towards the face. By contrast, if the cauda equina (nerve roots/peripheral nervous system) is involved then the resultant neurological picture is of a lower motor neurone lesion with precisely the opposite effect – reduced or absent reflexes and very low floppy tone, and no plantar responses.

The past 30 years has seen the increasing application of operative treatment in the management of spinal injuries just as we have seen in the management of limb injuries. Thirty years ago, or even 20 years ago, doctors looking after trauma patients tended to prescribe plaster of Paris immobilisation or traction, pulling on the leg with pins transfixing the bone below the fracture and then applying weights to counter muscle pull. We saw young adult males, for example, lying in traction with a steel pin through the shin bone just below the knee and weights applied to pull against the muscles of the thigh to control a fractured femur and such an individual might lie in bed for no less than 2 or even 3 entire months. The result was uncertain and while the majority might heal solidly, many did not heal satisfactorily or healed with an unacceptable degree of bending. Clearly, the older a patient is and being forced to lie in bed for 2 months, the higher the complication rate of so doing which would include blood clots in the legs (*deep vein thrombosis*, DVT) possibly going to the lungs to cause death (*pulmonary embolism*) as well as being *out of action* for a considerable period of time. Modern treatment protocols for limb injuries are that, with very few exceptions, it is highly advisable that these tubular long bones are fixed by the way of a nail passed down the marrow cavity (Fig. 6.7). The union rate is higher,

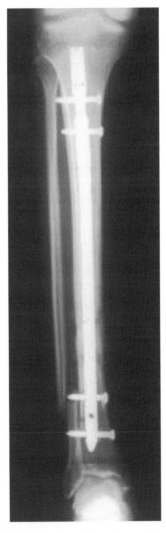

Fig. 6.7 This tibial fracture has been fixed with an intramedullary nail. It is difficult to break a bone without getting it fixed these days!

the alignment is virtually perfect, and the patient can be mobilised forthwith. Anything but a very physical occupation can be returned to in a matter of a few weeks or months rather than the categorical year that we used to prognosticate following a straightforward femoral fracture.

A similar trend has occurred in the management of spinal injuries and internal fixation is all the while being increasingly prescribed. Clearly, simple anterior wedge compression fractures are far too benign to warrant surgical consideration. What we are really trying to determine is the *stability* of the fracture. Burst fractures involve principally the squashing down of the vertebral body (the house) with sparing of the roof and although the appearances, particularly on any scans carried out, can look fairly daunting, there really is no reason to prescribe surgical intervention at least from the point of view of stability. Scans very often show that there is a piece of bone pushing backwards into the spinal cord (Fig. 6.4) but research has clearly shown that it is at the moment of injury when the cream of the meringue shocks the spinal cord that imparts the energy of paralysis and the appearances of a bit of cream indenting the spinal cord afterwards has no significant neurological effect. Seat-belt injuries that are through bone are inherently stable because the shark's teeth interdigitate on reduction to provide stability. Of course a seat-belt injury through disc endplate junction and posterior joint is less stable but nonetheless urgent surgery is not required, rather the patient would be followed up and if, on the occasions when ligaments do not heal in this situation, stabilising surgery can be carried out. The idea that you treat the whole for only a smallish part must be untenable particularly as there is an appreciable complication rate from tackling spinal injuries surgically.

It is really fracture–dislocations which are inherently unstable and merit consideration for prompt surgical treatment. Three scenarios present themselves as urgent reasons for surgical treatment. Most spinal injuries can be regarded as stable for nursing care if lying in bed and log-rolled appropriately. Log-rolled means that torso and pelvis are moved as one so that there is no tendency to cause spinal displacement. However, if the patient has multiple injuries and requires, say, surgical treatment of limb injuries and being placed in an unstable position on an operating table then clearly it would be advisable for the unstable spinal injury to be fixed first (Fig. 6.6). If the patient had a head injury with cerebral irritation and was thrashing around, surgical stabilisation would be very advisable. Finally, if the degree of displacement was such that the two ends of the spinal column were not in contact (total dislocation) then reduction and surgical stabilisation is the only way to stabilise the spinal column. Over and above these three critical indications, surgical treatment is not mandatory.

For 50 years or more spinal injury treatment centres, like Stoke Mandeville, pioneered and developed by Sir Ludwig Guttman, have expertly managed unstable spinal injuries without surgical help at all. By attention to the chest, the urinary tract and the skin, as well as log-rolling and reduction of the injury gradually in bed (postural reduction) they not only achieved just as good results as surgery could have done but also by treating the patient in a holistic fashion achieved life expectancies not significantly different from normal individuals. To the astonishment of the Guttmans of this world who were bringing spinal injury treatment centres to each health region, surgeons began to tackle these injuries by way of operations, such as laminectomy which, of course, very often made the patient worse. In a burst fracture, for instance, it is the lamina and posterior part of the spine, which is the only stabilising structure and its removal at surgery could be entirely predicted to cause more harm than good. Surgeons continued shooting themselves in the foot over the next two or three decades in the erroneous belief that an anatomical reduction was required rather than mere stability. Moreover, even in unstable spinal injuries with total paralysis, patients treated non-surgically can generally get into a wheelchair at about 6 weeks whereas following surgery this period of time may be reduced to 2 weeks. Therefore, what we are really talking about is an apparent gain of 4 weeks, which may pale into insignificance if the patient then has to spend 30 or more years in a wheelchair. Whatever treatment method is adopted, it is essential that the spine not be divorced from the remainder of the patient and in particular the paralysed individual must have the global treatment excellence of the spinal injury treatment centre.

The compelling appearance of bone in the spinal canal in burst fractures continually drives surgeons to *decompress* the spinal canal, which is akin to shutting the gate after the horse has bolted because the damage to the spinal cord has been done already at the instantaneous moment of energy application. The burst fracture with no neurological dysfunction can just as well be treated with a few days of bed rest until the local pain has subsided and then can be mobilised with a simple brace to maintain the spine's natural lateral profile and thus a reduced position. Such a brace would only be required for about a 6-week period. In addition, it takes some time to recover from major spinal surgery and, therefore, the real effect of surgery is to reduce by a bit the period of 6 weeks in the brace. The complications of infection, metalwork breakage and neurological damage from the operation itself have to be weighed against a few weeks in a brace and, therefore, it must be the case that a proper *risks and rewards* discussion should be carried out with the patient beforehand.

Miscellaneous Spinal Conditions

CHAPTER 7

INTRODUCTION

This short section, while not being so directly relevant to medico-legal matters, completes the clinical review of spine pathologies, which the spinal surgeon may be asked to address and indicates the wide variety of pathological conditions, which make up the clinical portfolio of the spinal surgeon. In addition, it gives the flavour of how far spinal surgery has come over the past two or three decades.

The great majority of low-back problems are mechanical in origin and, therefore, the patient is going to be less symptomatic, when resting than when active. Night pain is not a feature of degenerative conditions but is the classical symptom of *bone destruction*. Therefore, it is important when taking a history from a back pain patient to ask specifically about night pain as this is a *red flag* warning for a worrying pathological process, such as tumour or infection. Being woken up several times and often having to pace the room at night in an attempt to obtain relief is the classical symptom of tumour (Fig. 7.1), whereas back pain, temperature and tenderness are the clinical triad diagnostic of infection. Indeed only infection and fresh injury produce spinal tenderness. Then many low-back conditions are associated with a degree of stiffness in the morning, which tends to wear off after a few minutes of being up and about. By contrast, inflammatory spinal arthritis (spondylitis) is characterised by *early morning stiffness*, which may go on for an hour or two and then recur later in the afternoon. Such a pattern of stiffness is typical of inflammatory arthritis. Moreover, this type of arthritis leads to spreading ossification of the ligaments and joints of the spine and so ever increasing loss of movement occurs until the whole spine may be quite rigid (ankylosis). Thus, the full name of the condition is *ankylosing spondylitis*. As with other types of inflammatory arthritis, such as rheumatoid disease, these patients bear their condition with great fortitude and are amongst the most grateful and compliant patients that orthopaedic surgeons have to deal with.

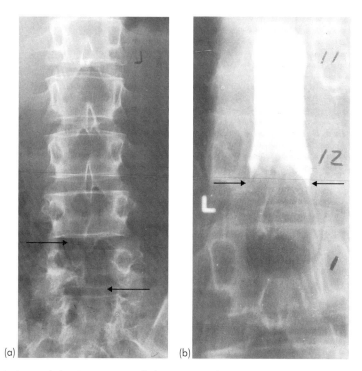

Fig. 7.1   This is an (a) AP X-ray and (b) AP myelogram of a young man of 25, who had complained of low-back pain and sciatica. (a) This figure shows that the man had undergone extensive low-back surgery including laminectomies at two levels (arrows) in the belief that the young man's problems were discogenic in nature. Had an adequate history been taken then one of the key symptoms that the young man complained of, namely, pain at night sufficient to wake him up and have him walk around the house, would have been elicited. (b) This figure shows that at the thoraco-lumbar junction (T12–L1) there is a complete block to the passage of myelogram dye due to an expanding intradural tumour (arrows).

TUMOURS

The great majority of spinal tumours are secondary malignant deposits from primary cancer elsewhere and common sites are lung, breast, prostate, kidney, gut and rarely thyroid gland. The history, physical examination and investigations are directed not only to the spine but to detect the likely primary site. While spinal secondaries tend to occur in an older age group this is tragically not always the case particularly with breast cancer. Naturally, treatment for widespread disease tends to be palliative, although on occasion removal of a primary kidney cancer can lead to regression or even disappearance of secondary deposits. There are two principal reasons for embarking upon spinal surgery and they are pain and paralysis. Malignant spinal pain can be devastatingly distressful being present every minute of the day and even worse at night. This is because the process of malignant bone destruction can be painful in its own right and this process can also lead to significant mechanical instability. While surgical excision is clearly going to be incomplete in that some malignant cells must be left behind, excision, grafting and stabilisation with metalwork are a merciful relief to the unfortunate patient and with adjuvant chemotherapy or radiotherapy can provide several years of symptomatic relief before the end. In this regard again, breast cancer can be very forgiving, while secondary lung cancer is so disappointing in its prognosis that surgery is seldom indicated.

Secondary malignant disease can also press on the spinal cord causing immobility and incontinence, which are also extremely distressing particularly if the natural history of the disease may mean survival for several years. Again spinal surgery has a very important role here and as most malignant spinal cord compression comes from the vertebral bodies at the front of the spinal cord with tumour extension upwards into the attic, the necessary surgical decompression should also be from the front. An individual nerve root compressed by a disc hernia can be safely decompressed from the back, but not the spinal cord, which occupies much of the spinal canal and could easily be damaged by manipulation and retraction to get round it to the front; moreover, the resultant bony deficit could not be grafted from a posterior approach. Such surgery might appear hazardous amongst the various thoracic and abdominal organs but there are no muscles attached to the front of the spine and once the lesion has been displayed there is excellent access for reconstruction. There is an increasing trend to do a *belt and braces* approach of front and back instrumentation and these procedures can, if necessary, be done under the one anaesthetic. Rather like the cauda equina syndrome, optimal results are achieved if paralysis is not complete at the time of surgery or if it has not been present for too long. Surgery may sound heroic but there are few more deserving cases than those with malignant spinal pain or impending paralysis and fewer more grateful patients in the whole spectrum of spinal surgery (Fig. 7.2).

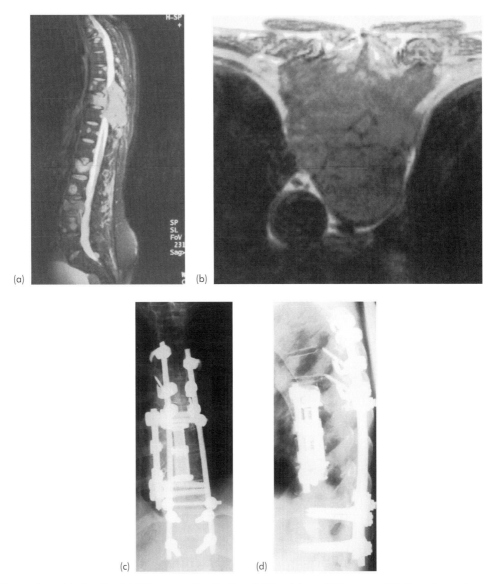

Fig. 7.2 (a) Sagittal MRI scan of a lady of 35 with a 2½-year-old daughter. A year previously she had undergone a radical mastectomy for breast cancer. The scan shows multiple spinal secondaries (areas where white has invaded bone) and in the mid-thoracic region there is extensive tumour formation both anteriorly and posteriorly, which compresses the spinal cord. (b) Axial MRI scan showing that the spinal cord is completely surrounded and encased in compressive tumour. Her legs were so weak that she could not walk and she required catheterisation for bladder instability. (c) AP and (d) lateral radiographs after extensive anterior and posterior decompression of the spinal cord and rebuilding of the spine with metalwork. Her neurological dysfunction recovered completely and she is still symptom-free and well 5 years later.

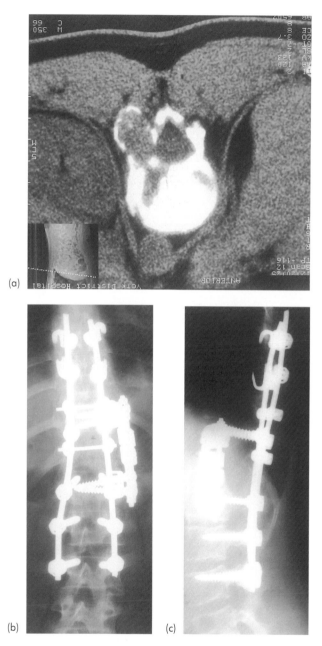

Fig. 7.3 (a) Axial MRI of the tenth thoracic vertebra of a 15-year-old boy with an unusual and aggressive benign tumour called a haemangioendothelioma. Note that there is dark coloured growth coming out of the left side of the vertebrae at the junction of the house and its roof. These growths can trun malignant and spread. (b) AP and (c) lateral radiographs after complete removal of the tenth thoracic vertebra, replacement with bone graft from the pelvis and supportive instrumentation front and back.

Benign tumours are much less common and tend to occur in adolescents or young adults, when the relevant cells are actively growing. Such lesions are very seldom malignant but do require complete removal otherwise recurrence is inevitable. This implies complete vertebrectomy carried out in a combined fashion front and back with the deficit made good harvesting graft material from the patient's own pelvis and securing it front and back with metalwork (Fig. 7.3).

INFECTION

The spine is a favourite site for infection to be deposited, when bacteria spread into the blood and cause infection (*septicaemia* or blood poisoning). Bacteria can come from several sources but the kidney and renal tract is a common primary site for acute infections, while tuberculosis (TB) tends to come from a primary focus in the lung. We have seen a great increase in more unusual opportunistic organisms with the rise in the number of individuals with AIDS or who are otherwise immuno-compromised. The triad of pain, temperature and tenderness is less obvious with tuberculous than acute infections and indeed TB may be relatively asymptomatic or entirely silent right up until paralysis.

Spinal infection – the diagnostic triad
- Back pain
- Temperature
- Tenderness

As symptoms can be so non-specific, even with acute spinal infections, it is more typical than not for presentation to be late or to masquerade as, for instance, abdominal or kidney infection. Therefore, delay in diagnosis, a very wide differential diagnosis, and even making the wrong initial diagnosis are more the rule than the exception. Except in the immuno-compromised patient the body does mount a response to the infection. Thus, there are blood markers, which are positive, such as a raised white cell count, plasma viscosity and C-reactive protein. Then the organism can be grown from the blood, while the spinal focus itself

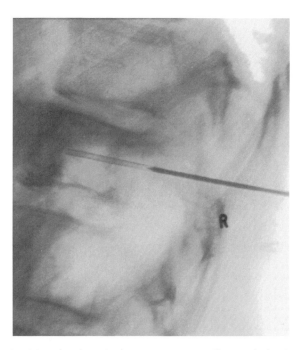

Fig. 7.4 Vertebral pathology can generally easily be biopsied with a percutaneous needle. This needle is inserted down the pedicle into the diseased vertebral body under X-ray control.

can be needle biopsied and the organism cultured (Fig. 7.4). It is important that material is sent to the pathology laboratory in addition to bacteriology as the diagnosis can be made microscopically; and this is particularly important, when the organism may have been suppressed by the previous administration of antibiotics making it difficult to culture.

The great majority of spinal infections can be treated conservatively with antibiotics to which the organism is sensitive, and because the spine can be painful and to minimise deformity, bracing for a few weeks is helpful. Sometimes no organism can be grown in which case antibiotics have to be empirically prescribed. To eradicate acute spinal infection a minimum of 6 weeks antibiotics requires to be administered, while it needs 6 months to a year if the infection is TB.

Most acute infections settle non-operatively but with TB it is common for patients to present with significant bone destruction, abscess formation, spinal instability, as well as paralysis (Fig. 7.5). Surgical treatment is along the same lines as that for

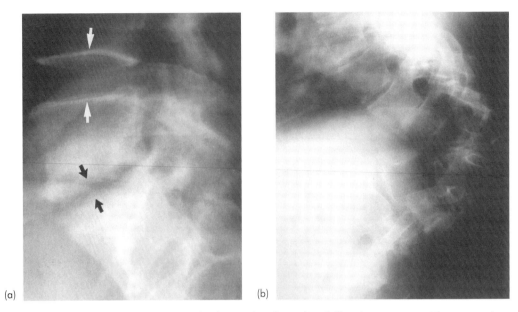

(a)   (b)

Fig. 7.5   (a) Bacterial infection of a lower lumbar disc following surgery. The organism must have entered during the operation. Note the moth-eaten and irregular appearance of the endplates of the adjacent vertebrae (black arrows). Compare that appearance with the normal endplates above which are sharply demarcated and regular (white arrows). This infection settled with antibiotics. (b) Untreated tuberculosis of the spine. As a result of bone and disc destruction the spine has progressively deformed and is now almost U-shaped. Surprisingly, perhaps, the patient had no evidence of paralysis.

tumour but the spinal cord compressed by spine infection is very much more forgiving than that if it is compressed by tumour.

ANKYLOSING SPONDYLITIS

This is a miserable combination of pain, stiffness and ever-decreasing spinal mobility. Nowadays, with anti-inflammatory drugs and physiotherapy a reasonable spinal shape can generally be preserved but more aggressive cases tend to become very round backed (kyphosis). This can be severe enough to prevent forward vision even using prismatic spectacles. Life then becomes a hazardous biological obstacle race and in such cases consideration should be given to surgical osteotomy (breaking and resetting the spine in a more erect position). The kyphosis tends to be in the thoracic region and that is where we do not like doing osteotomies because the spinal canal is

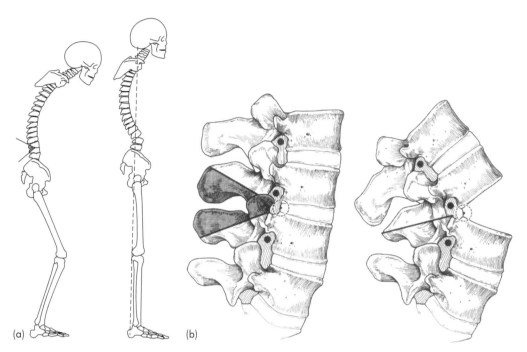

Fig. 7.6 Ankylosing spondylitis is a condition that you do not want to get. (a) The spine gradually ossifies and bends progressively further forward. Eventually, some patients cannot see anything but the ground and life becomes a worrying biological obstacle race. After osteotomy the spine is straighter and the patient can see forwards. (b) A wedge of bone is taken away from the back of the lumbar spine. From McMaster M. Surgery for ankylosing spondylitis. In: Operative Spinal Surgery (1991). Eds Torrens MJ, Dickson RA. Churchill Livingstone. Edinburgh & London.

small and is nearly filled with the very sensitive thoracic spinal cord. Accordingly, if thoracic kyphosis is high, we carry out our osteotomy at the junction of neck and thoracic spine where the canal is bigger, whereas if the kyphosis is lower then we perform the osteotomy in the upper-lumbar spine just below the spinal cord at the beginning of the cauda equina (Fig. 7.6). We carry out MRI scanning to determine at what level the end of the spinal cord is (usually the junction of L1 and L2). The higher osteotomy would be carried out at the C7/T1 level just below where the vertebral arteries enter the sides of the spine and are conveyed upwards into the head. Interference with the vertebral artery could give rise to a serious stroke and, therefore, operating below the C6 level avoids that complication.

Notwithstanding careful planning the complication list is long and important. The osteotomy is carried out in closing wedge fashion with the apex of the wedge in front of the dura so that when the wedge is closed the neurological tissue should not be stretched. Nonetheless, there is always a risk of nerve damage/paralysis. The aorta can also be stretched and this catastrophic complication can be fatal. In ankylosing spondylitis, the joints that the ribs make with the spine, so as to allow the chest to expand and contract with respiration, are commonly fused allowing no chest movement at all, respiration being achieved by upward and downward movements of the diaphragm, which is the muscle separating the chest from the abdomen. Accordingly, chest complications are not uncommon. Due to the markedly abnormal lateral profile of the ankylosing spondylitis neck, it can be very difficult to pass the anaesthetic tube beyond the larynx. This can sometimes be carried out successfully using a fibre-optic light source on a laryngoscope but it is not uncommon to have to carry out a preliminary tracheostomy. Although there seems to be no problem in forming bone with ankylosing spondylitis patients, as that is the underlying pathology, nonetheless, bone quality is often poor and metalwork can cut out of soft bone. External immobilisation with a brace or halo-cast is a necessary adjunct. Clearly, a careful risks and rewards discussion with the patient is crucial before embarking upon this type of surgery and one should have already gone through one's learning curve before taking these sorts of cases on. Fortunately, in some cases, there is concomitant hip arthritis and such hips tend to adopt a flexed position before they stiffen. Therefore, carrying out bilateral total hip replacements in such cases can itself make the patient erect and obviate the need for spinal surgery.

In addition to the ankylosing spondylitis bone being soft, there are two other very important mechanical matters in this condition. As the protective effect of a linked chain (movement occurring by contributions from many joints) is progressively lost so the spine's ability to shock absorb is drastically curtailed with the result that fractures occur much more readily with much less force than the normal spine and, moreover, once fractured, the loss of mobile joints above and below means there are long *lever arms* so that the ankylosing spondylitis fracture is much more vulnerable to displacement. Thus, while an unstable injury to a normal spine can be managed non-operatively by *log-rolling* (moving the patient as a whole to minimise displacement at the injury site) comparable injury in an ankylosing spondylitis spine may readily displace inducing paralysis. Accordingly, early surgical stabilisation has an important role in management.

Then, for whatever reason, one or more spinal joints may fail to stiffen and ossify, thus, providing a *stress-riser* (focal point of weakness) for the long lever arms to act upon. Surgical stabilisation of these *pseudarthroses* (failures of fusion) may be required.

SCOLIOSIS

Again, scoliosis is not of great relevance to personal injury litigation but is a concerning matter in the medical negligence field for both patient and surgeon. This is also of historical interest in that it was the scoliosis surgeons pioneering and developing spinal instrumentation techniques to correct spinal deformities in children that led to the application of similar metalwork systems to many other spinal pathologies as we have just seen. When the spine is viewed from the front or back it is supposed to be straight and if it is not then there is a lateral curvature of the spine, which we refer to as *scoliosis*. If one leg is a bit shorter than the other, a not all that uncommon occurrence, then unless one wants to point north–north-east one develops a secondary or compensatory scoliosis in the lumbar spine bringing the head up straight (Fig. 7.7). Such a scoliosis is unimportant and does not progress out of proportion with the underlying leg length inequality. Such a scoliosis is called *non-structural* (for no obvious semantic reason).

By contrast, scoliosis can appear for a variety of reasons and be progressive and self-perpetuating. Such scolioses nearly always have a twist to them as well and can produce nasty looking rib or loin humps. These progressive types of scoliosis are called *structural scoliosis*.

There are several different causes of structural scoliosis but by far the most common is called *idiopathic* scoliosis (idiopathic being the Greek for self-generating). Idiopathic scoliosis occurs in otherwise entirely normal children, whose spinal column has decided to buckle during growth. By contrast, non-idiopathic scolioses occur in association with another musculo-skeletal problem, for instance cerebral palsy (the neuromuscular control

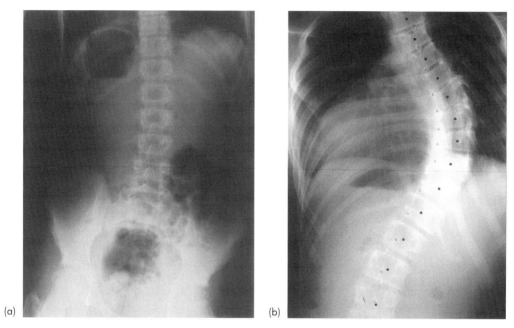

(a)   (b)

Fig. 7.7   (a) This is a standing frontal film showing a pelvic tilt because the legs are of unequal length. A secondary lumbar scoliosis develops bringing the head up straight. This is non-structural scoliosis. (b) By contrast, structural scoliosis has the spine straight at top and bottom but bending and buckling and twisting in the middle. This is a potentially progressive condition with growth.

of the spine is defective) or congenital scoliosis (the child was born with a congenital misshapen vertebra, which can be the central keystone for progressive deformity with growth).

There are three important issues in the management of a scoliosis case – organic health, shape and function. With regard to organic health, what is fundamentally important is when the scoliosis develops. Should there be a significant thoracic scoliosis (in the chest portion of the spine) during the first 2 or 3 years of life then this can seriously impede lung development and produce heart and lung morbidity and mortality in early adult life. If the deformity develops after the age of 5, however, there is no such risk (Fig. 7.8).

There are, in effect, two types of early onset progressive scoliosis that can give rise to organic ill health and they are *infantile idiopathic scoliosis* and *progressive congenital scoliosis*. A degree of scoliosis commonly occurs just after birth and, fortunately, the great majority resolve spontaneously. This tends to be in

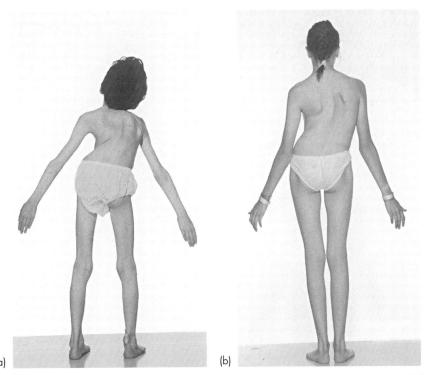

(a) (b)

Fig. 7.8 (a) Infantile progressive scoliosis. This 4-year-old boy has a very deformed chest and will have heart and lung problems in later life. (b) Adolescent idiopathic scoliosis: a matter of appearance and deformity only.

the normal birth weight, normally developing infant. However, the low birth weight, floppy baby not going through its milestones as fast as it should may not be able to resist a progressive scoliosis, which can have a catastrophic effect on the developing heart and lungs.

Fortunately, infantile progressive idiopathic scoliosis can, in many cases, be halted in progression or even straightened by the application of mini-plaster jackets, moulded as they are drying, carried out under a light general anaesthetic. Casts are changed every few months until about the age of 4 when growth rate flattens out.

Congenital anomalies of the spine

Progression can be very rapid in some. Unfortunately, progressive congenital scoliosis does not respond as favourably to cast

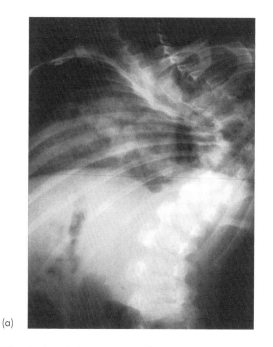 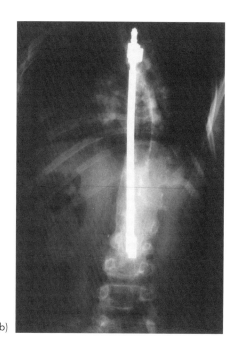

(a)   (b)

Fig. 7.9   (a) AP X-ray of a severe infantile progressive scoliosis. (b) Eight years after "growing" instrumentation. This rod has been lengthened or changed every 6–12 months to allow the back of the spine to continue growing. Very good control of this curve has been maintained and cardio-pulmonary complications mitigated.

management. Therefore, for the infantile progressive scoliosis that has not responded to cast treatment and for the very progressive congenital case surgery is necessary, although a daunting prospect. The fundamental problem of progressive scoliosis is that the front of the spine grows faster than the back and anterior spinal growth must be checked by anterior (through the chest) surgery. Then because the back of the spine relatively undergrows, it should be allowed to grow for as long as possible. Metalwork (hooks and rods) are attached to the spine to splint it and help it grow straighter. It can be lengthened as the child grows and so we call this the *growing instrumentation* (Fig. 7.9).

Adolescent idiopathic scoliosis

By far the commonest scoliosis that we treat is during adolescence, when spinal growth is rapid. As girls grow faster and earlier than boys their spines are more prone to buckling and we probably operate 10 times more girls than boys.

Importantly, this later onset scoliosis is not associated with any significant organic health problems because the lungs are already fully developed although bigger deformities can have extremely distressing social and psychological deprivation and dysfunction. Therefore, the effect of a significantly asymmetric torso should not be underestimated.

As the problem is one of appearance and deformity, it is very much the opinion of the patient and family (rather than the surgeon) that matters. The essential point with regard to adolescent idiopathic scoliosis is whether the deformity is acceptable or not. With adolescent growth, the deformity can change and what was acceptable at one stage may well become unacceptable a few years later. The spine grows until the early 20s and, therefore, unacceptability may not occur until then or even later.

The necessary treatment paradigm is fairly straightforward. If the deformity is acceptable then we should prevent it becoming unacceptable and if the deformity is unacceptable then we should make it acceptable and keep it acceptable until the spine has stopped growing. This, however, is more easily said than done. Unfortunately, non-operative treatment, generally wearing a torso brace, has been very disappointing, certainly not being able to straighten a buckling spine, nor have clinical trials shown an ability to prevent progression. Only major surgical intervention can significantly improve or straighten a bent spine but not without potentially serious complications.

This is where the scoliosis surgeon has to exercise his judgement to the limit, see the patient again and again, provide responsible counselling until such time as a decision is made as regards unacceptability and surgical treatment so that the only decision that can be made is the right one.

Fortunately, modern day surgical techniques do effect very good corrections. Operative treatment is by way of *instrumentation*, which straightens the spine, and maintenance of the correction is by what we call a *spinal fusion* whereby the entire curve, having been straightened, is fused solid rather like a fracture so that it cannot deform with subsequent growth (Fig. 7.10).

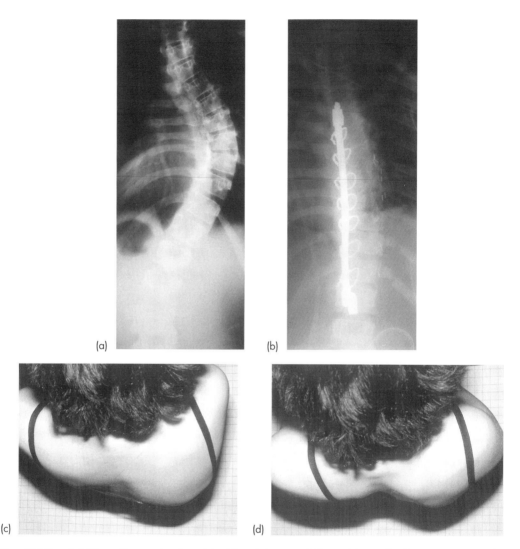

Fig. 7.10   (a) PA radiograph of a girl with adolescent idiopathic scoliosis pre-operatively. (b) After instrumentation and fusion showing an excellent correction. (c) The marked rib hump before surgery. (d) The excellent correction after surgery.

Arguments against this strategy in terms of making the spine stiff and stopping it from growing thereby stunting growth are quite unfounded. Untreated, the patient would be more bent and, therefore, shorter. An immediate benefit of surgery is, therefore, an instant increase in height of sometimes 2 in. or even more. Furthermore, these curves are very stiff because of the asymmetric shape of the vertebrae produced by uneven growth. Therefore, the true consideration is conversion of a bent stiff spine into a straighter stiff spine.

Each case is very individual mainly because of a different perception of what is, or is not, acceptable. Looking at X-rays and even looking at patients is not helpful in this regard. A 40° curve to one girl and family may be entirely acceptable, whereas a 40° curve to another might be so unacceptable as to produce serious psychological dysfunction.

By far the most important complication is paralysis and this is where the treatment of scoliosis differs so hugely from most other spinal disorders. We have a healthy and much loved teenage girl with a nasty deformity and the result should be correction or a very considerable improvement and the last thing we want to have is a paraplegic patient. Idiopathic scoliosis is generally so flexible that any stretching of the spine and spinal cord is well tolerated and so paralysis really should not be an issue, although the rather poor literature on this subject would suggest that the paralysis rate for idiopathic scoliosis might be something like one in 200. It certainly should not be higher. Real risks of paralysis in scoliosis surgery concern deformities, which are much more stiff, and also with congenital abnormalities within the spinal canal itself, thus, tethering the spinal cord and not making it amenable to a change in spinal shape.

Safety does, however, start before surgery and, now that we have MRI, scanning can be carried out to make sure the spinal cord is normal to begin with. During surgery itself, electrophysiological spinal cord monitoring is very helpful and here the patient is stimulated at one end of the spinal cord and at the other end the responses are picked up and displayed on what looks like an ECG machine. Any significant alteration in the wave pattern tells us that the spinal cord does not like what we are doing and allows us to stop straightaway and mitigate neurological loss. If metalwork has been inserted then this must be de-tensioned or removed as fast as possible. The point of electrophysiological monitoring is that after we put metalwork in the spine we may spend an hour or two doing a spinal fusion and perhaps resetting the ribs so that when the patient wakes up, may be 3 h later with paralysis, we have not wasted valuable time. Thus, unfavourable electrophysiological responses during surgery allow us to take remedial action as soon as possible. Alternatively, a "wake-up" test can be performed. The anaesthetic is lightened after instrumentation has been inserted to the point, where the patient can hear and understand the command to "wiggle your toes". If that is seen to be done satisfactorily then it means a normally functioning spinal cord between head and feet. The test is easy to perform and not remembered by the patient. Post-operatively, it is mandatory that the patient be monitored as regards neurological function in the legs for the first few days.

The treatment of neuromuscular scolioses is to aid function. When the spinal guy ropes do not work properly then the spine can sag and the non-walker can begin to fall out of their wheelchair or have to use their hands to prop themselves up depriving them of their normal prehensile function. Accordingly, surgery to prop them up may well be indicated. A good example of this would be the unfortunate boy with muscular dystrophy. All such patients will develop a scoliosis as their disease progresses threatening sitting stability. Spinal surgery, by providing a straighter erect firm spine, not only releases the hands but also improves quality of life, and chest function, and there is some evidence that it also prolongs life. The whole of the thoraco-lumbar spine requires to be instrumented (Fig. 7.11). Bleeding can be a problem and in some series, there is a 10% mortality rate. Clearly this has to be balanced against the potential benefits of surgery.

This completes this short additional section about the various spinal conditions, which spinal surgeons have to address on a daily basis and also hopefully indicates the sort of knowledge base, which only a spinal surgeon can draw upon when providing expert medico-legal spinal evidence. It certainly is a unique experience and not one that other health care professionals are exposed to.

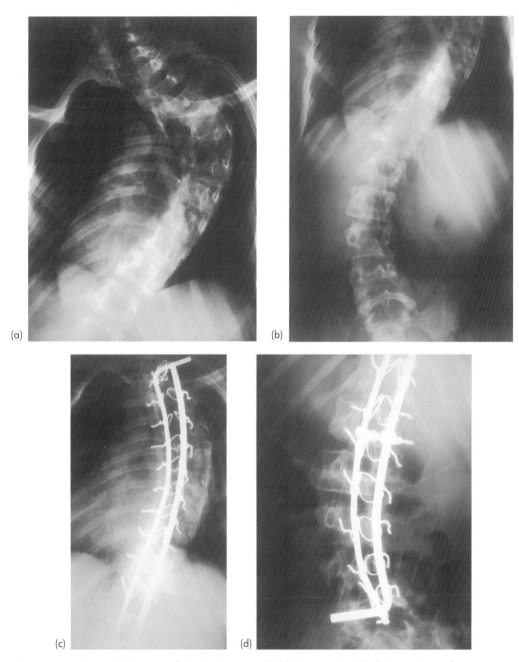

(a)

(b)

(c)

(d)

Fig. 7.11   Frontal X-rays of the (a) top and (b) bottom half of the spine of a teenage boy with muscular dystrophy who was falling out of his wheelchair. Frontal X-rays of the (c) top and (d) bottom half of the spine after full-length spinal instrumentation. This led to restoration of sitting stability and markedly improved function.

Back Pain and Litigation

INTRODUCTION

Those of us in reasonable health and full-time well-paid employment in the medical and legal professions do not, perhaps, realise how fortunate we are. By contrast, to a young bread winner with a family to support and a mortgage and other financial responsibilities and looking forward to enhanced security in the future, a severe injury resulting in significant symptoms as well as an inability to continue working is a catastrophic event. What would we do if it happened to us and how would we cope physically, emotionally and financially? Clearly, financial compensation from a genuine accident-related disability is entirely appropriate and well deserved, but it is no substitute for normality.

We have always been, and will remain, staunch supporters of the concept that an individual who is damaged deserves compensation. That is why compensation for damages is entirely valid, but such damages do seem to be often unfairly distributed.

THE EXPERT WITNESS

Experts involved in trying to help the medico-legal process should, we think, know something about the matter in hand and demonstrate reasonable clinical experience. Orthopaedic surgeons deal with the surgical aspects of all hard parts of the body, the bones and joints, and the muscles, tendons, ligaments and nerves that work them; that is, all bar the contained soft organs. The last 20 or 30 years have seen considerable subspecialisation because of the extraordinary developments that have taken place over this period in terms of both knowledge and clinical practice (e.g. in total joint replacement and spinal instrumentation). A modern day orthopaedic spine surgeon would not be competent to address a matter to do with a knee replacement or indeed a knee injury, while an orthopaedic radiologist would not opine as an expert about a chest X-ray, although he may know quite a lot about it.

The medico-legal process has burgeoned in recent years to the point where all sorts of health care professionals are getting involved but should not necessarily be regarded as being anything more than medical witnesses-of-fact. It is not easy to keep up with even the relevant spinal and radiological journals, let alone more general ones, and so medical expertise really ought to be much more stringently categorised. This has hugely important ramifications. The production of the medical report requires the taking of a history (asking questions of a patient), performing a physical examination, assessing X-ray appearances and reports thereof as well as often going through rain forests of documentation before a final opinion can be put forward. A general surgeon or physician's understanding of spine scan reports would be minimal, while their interpretation of the appearances of the films themselves would be frankly dangerous just as a spine surgeon's view of a CT scan of the abdomen would be as ridiculous to know about as to commission in the first place. Even a spinal surgeon's view of a spinal scan should be taken with more than a pinch of salt because the last decade has seen a huge multiplication in the number of spinal scans performed, the clinical nuances thereof and very importantly the accompanying literature underpinning it. Spinal surgeons who say they would always be prepared to take a patient to the operating theatre without discussing the scans with an experienced spinal radiologist are not exhibiting best practice.

A recurring and crucial theme in medical reports and in evidence in court concerns what is or is not an *appropriate* clinical response for a given condition. Experienced doctors in their particular field are able to establish in their own mind what is appropriate for a particular medical condition and axiomatically what is not appropriate. Acquisition of this essential core clinical information by seeing lots of patients, supplemented by awareness of what is happening elsewhere from attending courses and reading the relevant literature constitutes best *evidence-based practice*. It does, therefore, seem extraordinary how so many different opinions about the spine and low-back pain in particular are afforded in the Courts of this land when such seemingly gross differences of opinion are so uncommon in our clinical practice; while medico-legal reports on spinal patients are compiled by doctors from a wide range of specialties, doctors from many fewer specialties actually treat such patients.

Perhaps a good way forward might be to require experts, as a matter of course, to include their C.V.'s in their reports and not in separate documents. This would have the effect of requiring the expert to attest to his belief in the truth of the contents of his C.V. as well as the facts and opinions recorded in his report. He could then be cross-examined on his C.V. as well as his report.

Incidentally the time to back up opinion with references is along with the substantive medical report. All too often this unfortunately doesn't happen and it is not at all uncommon even as late as Woolfian joint statement stage for a host of "abstracts" (a few summary lines and a miserable fraction of the full paper, with all the necessary data and analysis to study missing downloaded from the internet at a touch of a button from a computerised database such as Medline) to be suddenly disclosed as if to confuse the medico-legal process rather as "chaff" sought to deflect radar signals in World War 2, as our more senior readers will readily remember. Such a practice does not befit the medico-legal process and the Court should firmly disallow it. More often than not, rather like the unindicated MRI scan, the litigation is not only not assisted but frankly hindered and always leads to delay. If you want to talk to your opposite number about a particular publication, then disclose the text in full and in good time. Not to do so is impolite and unhelpful and thus not "good medical procedure".

All individuals who have a special interest in the management of back pain should be allowed to have their say, although only spinal *surgeons* should opine about the *surgical* aspects of back-pain management. So-called clinical expertise from a non-practising individual should be disallowed and that means anyone who has not been in active clinical management of back pain in, say, the past 2 years. We all know how quickly clinical touch can be lost. Only experts should be allowed to be expert witnesses and expert witnesses should only be experts. This means experience. Talking to claimants is not experience; but talking to patients is.

- Only experts should be expert witnesses.
- Expertise means clinical experience.
- Talking to claimants is not experience.

Fortunately, the implementation of the civil procedure rules (CPR) on 26th April 1999, which binned the old regime in favour of the Courts themselves actively managing cases, should help greatly in many regards, including the matter of expert witnesses. Lawyers, of course, will know the ins and outs of CPR backwards but some orthopods, or other doctors, may not in which case a dip into the new edition of "Medicolegal reporting in orthopaedic trauma"[1] by Foy and Fagg is recommended (Foy and Fagg sound more like a firm of Solicitors than a pair of Consultant Orthopaedic Surgeons!). Two of the introductory four chapters are written by Solicitors and provide a lot of useful information about the medico-legal process and in particular the role of the expert witness. The duties and responsibilities of expert witnesses were usefully set out in the more recent case of Ikarian Reefer (1993) 2 Lloyds Rep 68.81 from which there was a plethora of expert evidence much of which offered little or no assistance! The Court endorsed Lord Wilberforce's comments in *Whitehouse v Jordan* and added that "if an expert had insufficient expertise or lacked information in a certain area then the expert must say so". Lord Wilberforce's use of the word *must* should make matters crystal clear.

ILLNESS BEHAVIOUR

The claimant's behaviour may be *appropriate* and in no way different from the 50 patients that come to our Monday spinal clinic or *inappropriate* with a clinical presentation, which is in marked contrast to our usual spinal patient with the exhibition of symptoms and signs not appropriate to our clinical experience with patients who have the same condition. As we expect honesty from our experts, we should also expect the same from claimants and perhaps a way forward is to suggest that a more detailed history be available by way of a statement prior to an examination that would form part of the claimant's evidence possibly on the basis of a questionnaire being supplied by the particular doctor examining. However, this would require a reform of CPR as matters stand.

Pilowsky[2] pointed out that this matter of abnormal illness behaviour goes back to the 1700s, when medical literature referred to this as being *hysteria* (an uncommon psychoneurosis with anaesthesia – you can stick pins in yourself with no apparent pain sensation!) or *hypochondriasis* (anxiety about one's health or morbid depression without real cause), both at that time thought to be the same condition. As qualified doctors, we do know what these words mean in the same way that we would know that our psychiatric colleagues would understand what we meant by spinal fracture or disc hernia.

Indeed, it is important to know what these basic different conditions mean so that we can understand when to refer for appropriate management without claiming any expert knowledge in the management of such cases, let alone purporting to be an expert witness thereupon.

Minds were polarised about this matter in the middle of the last century when Henry Miller, a neurologist from the north east, opined that many individuals with the so-called post-concussional syndrome were *malingerers* and that their symptoms were either invented or exaggerated. It is often thought, even in legal circles where the meaning of words is so important, that malingering means complete invention of disability. This is not so. The Oxford dictionary definition of to malinger is to *pretend or exaggerate illness in order to escape duty or work*.

> Malingering is the pretence or exaggeration of illness in order to escape duty or work

Miller's view that you were either perfectly normal on the one hand, or malingering on the other, rather set the cat amongst the pigeons and, not surprisingly, some common sense fairly shortly thereafter began to prevail, and the concept of a range of *illness behaviour* soon emerged. There is a spectrum of human response to a medical problem from, shall we say, stoicism at one end of the spectrum to what can be referred to as *abnormal illness behaviour* at the other. Meanwhile, as we move through this spectrum, we would encounter somebody with *normal illness behaviour* in that some anxiety and depression combined with heightened clinical responses might not be unexpected in someone with 5 years, say, of fairly severe low-back pain. At the abnormal illness behaviour end of the spectrum would be someone, whose responses are quite inappropriate and out of proportion to the underlying problem.

Pilowsky[2] wrote wisely about this subject pointing out that the nub of this matter was *the diagnostic problem presented by the patient with physical complaints for which no adequate organic cause can be found.* At the time of his article in the late 1960s, he noted that there was a large number of diagnostic labels, for example *functional illness, functional overlay, hysteria, hysterical overlay, conversion reaction, psychophysiological reaction, somatisation reaction, hypochondriasis, invalid reaction, neurasthenia, psychogenic regional pain, psychosomatic, psychological invalidism, malingering, Munchausen's syndrome and organic neurosis!* He said that *non-psychiatrists are certainly not entirely to blame for this unsatisfactory situation since psychiatrists have for many years been equally uncertain in this area.* Of course, there would be obviously no reason why a patient with advanced cancer should not show abnormal illness behaviour but the title of his article *Abnormal illness behaviour* focused quite clearly on the difficulties arising in the diagnosis of patients who complain of physical symptoms in the absence of an adequate organic cause, in particular regarding unexplained pain. Despite whatever diagnostic label one would wish to attach, he pointed out that *what appears to require emphasis is that the doctor is conveying his belief that although the patient expects to be regarded as physically ill, this is not justified by the objective pathology present.* He brought into the equation two important and related sociological concepts concerning illness – *the sick role* and *the notion of illness behaviour.* It was described that *the sick role is a partially and conditionally legitimate state – the sick person is granted the role provided that he accepts that it is an undesirable one and recognises his obligation to co-operate with others for the purpose of getting well as soon as possible.* Furthermore, this individual's *disability and incapacity are not regarded as something for which he can be held responsible and are, therefore, not considered to be his fault.* However, it was strictured that *clearly the sick role may not be granted if there appears to be inadequate evidence for the presence of a disease process which would justify that role.*

As regards the second relevant concept, that of illness behaviour, this was defined as *the ways in which given symptoms may be differentially perceived, evaluated and acted (or not acted) upon by different kinds of person.* The common factor underlying illness behaviour was *that the doctor's belief was that although the patient wanted to be regarded as ill, the objective pathology did not justify this.* Pilowsky phrased this as *the doctor does not believe that the patient's objective pathology entitles him to be placed in the type of sick role he expects for the reasons which he claims it. If the patient is uninfluenced by the doctor's explanation of what he believes to be the problem and the way in which it should be managed, the doctor may then reasonably conclude that the patient is manifesting abnormal illness behaviour.*

Pilowsky added that the question of *motivation involves a spectrum from totally unconscious seeking of the dependency gratifying and guilt allaying aspects of the sick role to the entirely conscious attempt to obtain financial compensation.* The approach to these individuals emphasised the need for careful evaluation of the organic component along with all other aspects.

This was a seminal point in time – the beginning of an understanding of illness behaviour and changing it from a one or the other position to a spectrum. This allowed one to start to appreciate the intricacies of these sorts of matters. The importance of this medico-legally is that this is not a black and white decision and it cannot be made by any person other than a doctor clinically experienced in this field, who can translate that experience into the medico-legal scenario. The notion that a spinal surgeon thought that the spinal patient behaved perfectly appropriately while the diabetologist claimed that the patient displayed abnormal illness behaviour is just as ludicrous as the spinal surgeon saying that a diabetic was over-reacting, when the diabetologist asserted that the patient's responses to diabetes were normal. Expert witnesses should be experts with considerable clinical experience in that area.

Although we are strong supporters of the concept of the injured person deserving compensation, we are equally opposed to the misuse of clinical medicine, spine surgery or radiological investigation for that purpose. In our experience, such misuse is widespread and common, particularly in the inappropriate requisition of MRI scanning which has no place in the medico-legal scenario.

Many claimants with back pain who end up in court have a clinical presentation never seen in back-pain clinics. The grimacing, huffing and puffing, standing up and sitting down every 10 min, and indeed being invited to do so by the judiciary, is something that does not occur in back-pain clinic waiting areas and one naturally wonders if this behaviour is learnt rather than spontaneous. Such behaviour is often considered *honest, reliable and non-exaggerated* by the court indicating that non-expert evidence and inexperience have prevailed. Indeed, we recently heard a judgement in a case, where the judge commented that because the claimant sat still throughout the day of trial she was not disabled, thereby illustrating the fact that the courts see and consider normal behaviour that is unnatural. There should be no place for empiricism in the medico-legal process.

Since the late 1960s, a lot of rhetoric has arisen about the subjects of illness behaviour in relation to the lumbar spine, and to back pain in the work place, and two individuals in particular have contributed very significantly in this regard – Prof. Gordon Waddell from Glasgow (illness behaviour) and Prof. Alf Nachemson from Gothenberg, Sweden (back pain in the workplace).

INAPPROPRIATE CLINICAL FEATURES

Waddell[3] started by looking at failed lumbar disc surgery following industrial injuries and examined more than 100 workman's compensation board patients in the Toronto area. The focus was mainly on repeat spine surgery. The diagnostic criteria of a prolapsed disc were of *a predominant complaint of sciatica, straight leg raising reduced by sciatica, presence of neurological abnormalities and a radiological image demonstrating a disc hernia at the level that fitted the clinical picture*. Three of these four were required to establish the presence of a surgically remediable disc hernia.

Diagnosis of a prolapsed disc

- Predominantly sciatica – sciatic pain much worse than back pain (disc surgery is nerve root decompression and will not reduce back pain)
- Straight leg raising reduced by sciatica only – not by back pain
- Neurological abnormalities – appropriate to the relevant nerve root
- Scan positive – showing interference with the right nerve root on the right side
- Do non-, or occasional, *spinal* specialists really know this?

Then, it was stressed that *an adequate conservative treatment programme was an essential prerequisite to surgery for pain and 3 months should be considered the minimum.* Of course, in those days bed rest was strictly observed and now we would not recommend that but try and emphasise mobility. Interestingly, one-third of patients with an initial diagnosis of prolapsed disc had only one or even none of the four criteria and a sixth had a spell of conservative treatment that fell far short of that just described. Sciatica recurring after a period of relief of at least 6 months or due to a disc prolapse at a new level gave a success rate comparable to the first operation but scarring, previous infection, failed fusion and adverse psychological factors precluded a good result.

Waddell found that by any criteria *these results for repeat back surgery for degenerative lumbar disc disease in compensation patients are bad* and the second operation should generally be regarded as the last chance. *Psychological factors should be given due consideration before reaching any decision as to operate and the presence of compensation undoubtedly alters these psychological and social aspects.* Waddell commented that *11 comparative reports suggest that the results of any form of treatment of low-back pain in compensation patients average one-third poorer than in non-compensation patients.* Therefore, in a substantial proportion of these individuals, desperation, duration of symptoms, a desire to help or a desire to *give the patient a chance* were not proper surgical indications leading to the statement that *there is no place for a blind philosophy of try, try and try again.* The key was selection of – *surgeon, patient, operation or withholding surgery.* Therefore, a very important point coming through was that surgeons were often persuaded to operate, and indeed regrettably still are, when the required clinical algorithm has not been strictly adhered to.

Waddell[4] then went on to evaluate a series of physical signs that appeared to have a predominantly non-organic basis that were described at the beginning of the 20th century following the introduction of the Compensation Acts and the development of medico-legal practice. As Pilowsky had indicated, these non-organic signs were interpreted initially as evidence of malingering, although with increasing psychological knowledge this appeared to be an over-simplification to the point where the signs were in danger of being discredited or ignored. A standardised group of five types of physical signs were developed and formed the basis for this and many other investigations.

Non-organic physical signs in low-back pain

- Tenderness
  - Superficial
  - Non-anatomic
- Simulation
  - Axial loading
  - Rotation
- Distraction
  - Straight leg raising
- Regional
  - Weakness
  - Sensory
- Over-reaction
  - Puffing, panting
  - Groaning, grimacing
  - Resisting

Tenderness in relation to physical disease is usually located close to a particular musculo-skeletal structure, while non-organic tenderness may be either superficial or non-anatomic (Fig. 8.1). Skin tenderness is neither a feature of lumbar spine pathology nor tenderness over a very wide area. Indeed, tenderness is only elicitable from three, or possibly four, underlying pathologies. With spinal infection, whose diagnostic triad is back-pain temperature and tenderness, tenderness is an essential feature. It is also common with fresh injury and is sometimes elicitable in severe inflammatory arthritis and tumours. Otherwise, the lower back is not tender and certainly not with degenerative disease of either disc or joint months or years after musculo-ligamentous strains.

Simulation refers to back pain being produced by *rotation of shoulders and pelvis* when, of course, the back itself is not being rotated (Fig. 8.2). *Axial loading* refers to gentle pressure over the dome of the head producing low-back pain, when the energy of such a load would be absorbed by the first cervical joint (Fig. 8.3).

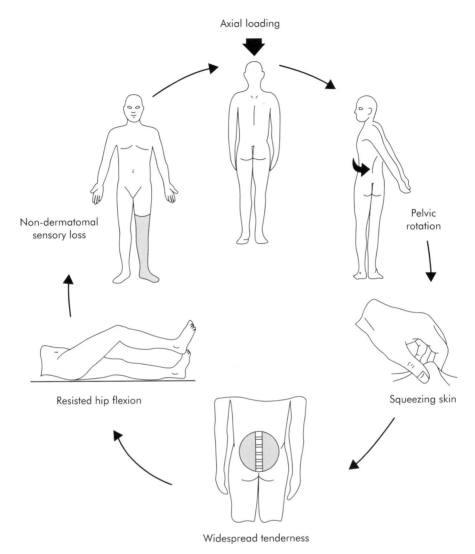

Axial loading

Non-dermatomal
sensory loss

Pelvic
rotation

Resisted hip flexion

Squeezing skin

Widespread tenderness

Fig. 8.1 Six inappropriate findings on examination. From Porter RW (1993). Management of Back Pain. Second Edition. Churchill Livingstone. Edinburgh & London.

Distraction testing refers to examining the patient supine and assessing the degree of straight leg raising (Fig. 8.4) and then finding that the patient can, for example, sit up on the examination couch with their legs out in front of them or sit on the examination couch with the knees flexed and then extend them to examine the foot reflexes. Sitting up is another good example of distraction in demonstrating the extent of lumbar spine movements. A complaint of only a few degrees of forward flexion

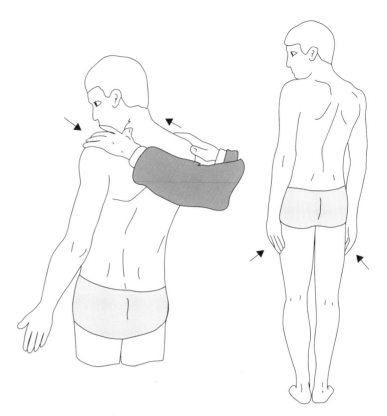

Fig. 8.2 Simulated rotation producing back pain is inappropriate.

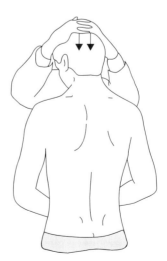

Fig. 8.3 Pressure on top of the head cannot produce low-back pain.

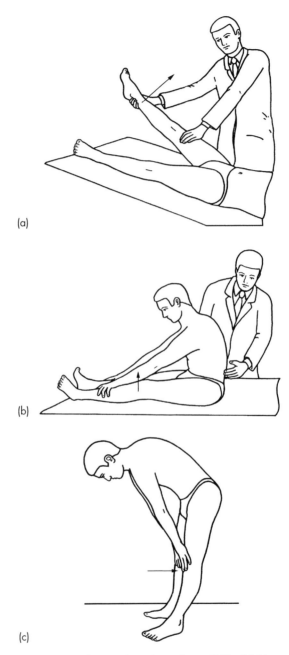

(a)

(b)

(c)

Fig. 8.4   (a) Straight leg raising is seemingly restricted at about 30°. (b) However, the patient can sit up on the examination couch with the legs extended in front of them indicating a positive distraction test and an inappropriate straight leg raising response. (c) If forward bending of the spine is restricted standing up but the patient can fully flex the spine sitting up on the examination couch (b) then this is another inappropriately positive distraction test.

being possible when standing up is not compatible with a full range of lumbar spine movement sitting with the legs extended out in front.

Then, *regional* disturbances include muscle weakness not explained on a neurological basis and in particular weakness without muscle wasting. Pain can sometimes be responsible for a bit of weakness but usually, with persuasion, normal power can be demonstrated. However, any significant degree of muscle weakness must be accompanied by wasting of that muscle because weakness is caused by wasting. Then, remembering our dermatomes, there are three fairly discrete dermatome distributions in the leg below the knee and finding, for instance, reduction or loss of sensation in a stocking distribution affecting, say, the whole of the leg below the knee (Fig. 8.1) or the whole of the lower extremity below the groin implies either a serious pathological process affecting the nerve roots L2–S4 inclusive, a most unlikely situation, or the presence of non-organic features.

Finally, *over-reaction* refers to disproportionate verbalisation, facial expression, muscle tremor, puffing and panting, sweating and in some cases the inability to undergo a satisfactory examination at all. In addition to increasing voluntary muscle tension and tremor, the neck and trunk may well be flexed upwards in protest at more than a few degrees of straight leg raising. Such flexion tensions the meninges which surround the nerve roots and are a diagnostic test for meningitis. Such flexion would make genuine radicular pain on straight leg raising far worse rather than better. It was stressed that isolated positive signs should not themselves be regarded as diagnostic but a finding of three or more of the five types was deemed clinically significant. It was concluded that *these non-organic signs were independent of, and separable from, the standard clinical science of physical pathology and that non-organic signs correlated with other clinical non-organic assessments. These non-organic signs should form part of a routine pre-operative screen to help identify patients who require detailed psychosocial assessment.* In other words, psychosocial factors were already known to be associated with a poorer clinical result following spinal surgery and this was an attempt to identify suitable signs by which such psychosocial dysfunction could be recognised, in the context of lumbar spine surgery, and trying to select patients in a much more precise fashion.

This particular paper began a lifetime's work by Waddell and his colleagues and it is important to appreciate that these non-organic physical signs were very selective, were used so that they could be scored and tested statistically as regards reproducibility and stability as well as being able to be correlated with standard psychological questionnaires. Such signs are necessarily only a part of the clinical examination phase of patient consultation, do not include all the physical signs that we elicit and exclude the clinical history, or the symptoms, of the complaint (Table 8.1).

It is this holistic evaluation that can only be carried out by a spinal specialist. As Waddell stated *all good clinicians use a clinical interview and examination not only to diagnose physical disease but also to learn about the patient and his or her response to illness.* Again the poor outcome from low-back surgery for compensation cases was emphasised.

Table 8.1 Symptoms as well as signs of abnormal illness behaviour.[5] Comparison of symptoms and signs of physical disease and abnormal illness behaviour in chronic low-back pain. From Waddell G, Bircher M, Finlayson D, Main CJ. Symptoms and signs: physical disease or illness behaviour? British Medical Journal 1984, 289: 740. Reproduced with permission from the BMS Publishing Group.

	Physical disease and normal illness behaviour	Magnified or inappropriate illness behaviour
Symptoms		
Pain	Localised	Whole leg pain, tailbone pain
Numbness	Dermatomal	Whole leg numbness
Weakness	Myotomal	Whole leg giving way
Time pattern	Varies with time	Never free of pain
Response to treatment	Variable benefit	Intolerance of treatment, emergency admissions to hospital
Signs		
Tenderness	Localised	Superficial, widespread, non-anatomical
Axial loading	No lumbar pain	Lumbar pain
Simulated rotation	No lumbar pain	Lumbar pain
Straight leg raising	Limited on distraction	Improves with distraction
Sensory	Dermatomal	Regional
Motor	Myotomal	Regional, jerky giving way
General response	Appropriate pain	Over-reaction

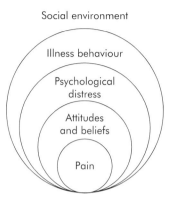

Fig. 8.5 Waddell's biopsycho/social model of low-back pain. From Waddell G (1996). Keynote Address for Primary Care Forum. Low Back Pain: A Twentieth Century Health Care Enigma. Spine; 21(24): 2820–2825.

Then this model of illness behaviour (Fig. 8.5) was taken further[6] and a mathematical relationship was developed between measured elements of illness behaviour and it was demonstrated that the most important psychological disturbance in low-back pain is emotional distress. By far the most powerful psychological influences were questionnaire measures of depression and bodily awareness, clinical measures of inappropriate symptoms and signs, and it was clearly shown that *there was no evidence of psychiatric illness either from psychological testing or during the psychologist's interview, confirming general clinical experience that referral of a chronic-pain patient to a traditional psychiatrist usually fails to elucidate any psychiatric explanation or help.*

This model was then tested as an improved basis for surgical decision-making in low-back disorders in a prospective way[7]. 185 patients who had undergone a number of different types of low-back surgery were evaluated over 2 years from surgical intervention and it was found that the physical outcome was entirely determined by physical fact, such as *accuracy of diagnosis of a surgically treatable lesion, operative findings, surgical procedure and avoidance of complications.* The most important psychological disturbance was *distress and abnormal illness behaviour that could affect surgical outcome indirectly if inappropriate illness behaviour led to inappropriate surgery and also directly affected subjective judgements of pain or disability by patient or observer.* Return to work was strongly influenced by additional occupational factors. They concluded that this model or concept of illness as proposed formed the basis of a fundamental reconsideration of clinical management and surgical decision-making in low-back disorders. Waddell concluded by saying that medicine has always recognised the need to treat the whole person – *holistic not in the sense of alternative medicine but simply as good clinical practice. The challenge facing medicine now is to put the art of medicine on to a sound scientific basis, to improve our treatment of patients to match our ever-increasing ability to treat disease. The goal is beyond dispute. The means lies in our concept of illness.*

The same patients were then assessed critically as regards outcome measures including return to work.[8] *Interestingly, despite the original criteria laid down for grading outcome as good, fair or poor, neither patient nor surgeon was influenced to any extent by whether or not surgery resulted in return to work. Conversely, return to work was determined to a surprisingly small extent by either the physical findings or the effect of surgery and was much more strongly influenced by social and work-related factors.* This supports clinical experience and explains why the proportion of patients returning to work varies so much. Ten years later, many other studies showed the same trend about return to work as we shall see more of later.

Then, Prof. Waddell[9] and the clinical psychologist Prof. Chris Main formulated the distress and risk assessment method (DRAM) as a simple patient classification to identify distress and evaluate the risk of poor outcome. Subjects were evaluated as regards distress and illness behaviour using a number of techniques including the modified somatic perception questionnaire (MSPQ), the modified Zung depression index, the inappropriate non-organic signs test and the inappropriate symptoms test, which comprise the key elements of the Glasgow illness model. As a result, four categories of patient were identified – type N (normal), no evidence of distress or abnormal illness behaviour, low on all scales; type R (at risk), patients showing slightly higher scores than N patients; type DD (distressed depressive), patients showing clear elevation on all variables; and type DS (distressed somatic), patients more elevated than type N patients but particular elevation on the MSPQ somatic awareness test. Then, following surgical intervention it was noted, for instance, that 13% of type N patients had a medium or high disability at follow-up compared with almost 70% of type DD or DS patients, giving a more than 5 times higher risk of a poor disability outcome for distressed patients. There was a clear increase in the percentages of poor outcomes with increasing levels of distress. The percentages of poor outcomes were approximately doubled in type R versus type N patients and 3–4 times as large in type DD or DS versus type N. *It was stressed that DRAM was a first stage screening procedure and neither a complete psychological assessment nor a test of malingering. It highlighted individuals, who required much more careful psychosocial assessment before facing the prospect of surgical intervention.*

It had already been pointed out about the evaluation of results of lumbar spine surgery that evidence of illness behaviour was not the be-all and end-all by any means, but rather that very few clinical investigations into the outcome of lumbar spine surgery patients were really assessed organically in any convincing way. It was strictured that *follow-up should be for a minimum of 3 years and include at least 80% and preferably 90% of the patients operated upon. This post-op assessment should be carried out by an independent observer and not by the operating surgeon.* Ideally, identical assessment should be carried out pre-operatively and at follow-up, although patients and observers appear to assess the outcome of surgery more on the end result rather than on any change resulting from surgery.

Then, some useful definitions followed[9] with pain being defined as an *unpleasant sensory and emotional experience associated with actual or potential tissue damage, or described in terms of such damage.* It was shown that *impairment and disability* are fundamentally different. *Impairment* is *any loss or abnormality of psychological, physiological or anatomical structure or function,* while *disability is the resulting diminished capacity for everyday activities in gainful employment or limitation of a patient's performance compared to a fit person of the same age and sex stemming from the above-mentioned impairment.* The fundamental distinction is that pain and disability are subjective being based on the patient's self-report, while physical impairment is an objective evaluation carried out by the physician.

Again this stresses the importance of lumbar spine matters being evaluated by lumbar spine surgeons/specialists. Then, of course, *illness and injury/disease* are two discretely different matters. *Illness* is *the subjective impression of being unwell* and may, of course, occur quite independently of any physical injury or disease. Meanwhile, *injury* or *disease* is a *pathological process,* which in turn may exist independently of illness, that is, produce no symptoms, such as high blood pressure (you can have a very pathologically elevated high blood pressure and no symptoms therefrom. You may get them in the future if the blood pressure is not controlled but you very often have no symptoms to begin with). These are fundamental and now well-established precepts of contemporary medical practice. In this regard, perhaps, the lumbar spine is a notable example, with very little evidence of illness from a wide range of seemingly important pathological processes.

> • Pain – unpleasant sensory and emotional experience associated with actual or potential tissue damage or described in terms of such damage
> • Impairment – loss or abnormality of psychological, physiological or anatomical structure or function
> • Disability – the resulting diminished capacity for everyday activities in gainful employment or limitation of a patient's performance from the above-mentioned impairment
> • Illness – the subjective impression of being unwell
> • Injury/disease – a pathological process

With all sorts of different health care professionals getting involved in back pain for all sorts of different reasons, it was entirely appropriate for Chris Main and Gordon Waddell[10] to recently update us on the behavioural responses to examination and reappraise the interpretation of non-organic signs. They stressed that these signs were associated with other clinical measures of illness behaviour and were not simply a feature of medico-legal presentations. They stated quite categorically that despite clear caveats about the interpretation of the signs, they had been misinterpreted and misused both clinically and medico-legally. *Behavioural responses to examination provide useful clinical information but need to be interpreted with care and understanding.* As Waddell originally indicated, *isolated signs should not be over-interpreted or indeed interpreted at all.* Meanwhile, multiple signs suggest that the patient does not have a straightforward physical problem. That psychological and non-physical factors also need to be considered was again restated. They further strictured that behavioural signs may be responses affected by fear and the context of recovery from injury (in this case surgery) and the development of chronic incapacity. They offered only a psychological *yellow flag* and not a complete psychological assessment. Behavioural signs are not on their own a test of credibility or faking. Again, and one cannot stress this often enough, the assessment of a lumbar spine patient is the responsibility of a lumbar spine specialist, and clearly, the presence of non-organic features can only be understood by one with an understanding of the organic features of a case.

A very common accompaniment of back-pain litigants is the walking stick, the pair of crutches and even the wheelchair. Apart from the patient with severe rheumatoid spinal disease, secondary cancer or spinal fracture–dislocation complicated by paralysis, it is difficult to envisage any physiological function for these aids and appliances and they are not prescribed in NHS practice with the possible exception of a walking stick for balance in, say, an elderly frail individual. Moreover, these aids and appliances are nearly always self-prescribed, they are certainly not necessary physically and their inappropriate usage does tend to result in the bizarre gait one so often sees, which in turn is very much more likely to perpetuate low-back problems rather than alleviate them. Nearly all low-back problems are mechanical and if there is a particularly symptomatic phase then rest by lying or sitting is infinitely more preferable to standing and bending. A preferred standing posture, or repetitive standing and sitting, would make a physical back problem worse rather than better and indicates another inappropriate response.

It is important to understand that these signs are but a part of the overall evaluation of the spinal patient. As Bannister[1] points out *"the medico-legal consultation is different. There are fewer fractures and more back and neck injuries than in clinical trauma practice. The history from the Claimant may be unreliable, while physical signs are more likely to be influenced by psychological overlay and therapeutic interventions are often less effective. If a treatable condition can be identified, this should be regarded as a bonus rather than an expectation. A description of onset of symptoms some months after the accident makes causation questionable*". As Mr Justice Ian Kennedy[1] stated "*by definition a condition is not an injury unless its presence is attributable to the accident*". Severity of symptoms is useful for future comparison and a pain analogue score of 0 (no pain) to 10 (the worst pain imaginable) allows progress to be assessed and gives some indication of the claimant's pain threshold. Bannister added that "*a claim of discomfort of 8–9 out of 10 for symptoms that does not merit analgesia suggests enhanced pain appreciation or exaggeration. Progress of symptoms, should be noted. Most skeletal trauma improves, then stabilises. Resolution of symptoms, followed by relapse months or years later, is recorded in the literature but is atypical*".

Bannister went on to point that "*while claimants describing chronic severe pain often take no medication stating that they don't like tablets and emphasising their stoicism, in clinical practice patients with severe hip or back pain usually discontinue medication only because of recognised side effects*". To the aforementioned list of inconsistent signs, Bannister adds that "*claims of inability to carry out manual work are inconsistent with dirt-ingrained fingers with thickened skin. The inability to flex the neck and back or raise the upper limb makes hair care and painting toenails physically impossible and a description of extreme depression with restricted mobility is generally inconsistent with an immaculate personal appearance. Over-reaction by movement at a speed more likely to cause pain is inconsistent with the presentation of pure organic disease*".

Physical signs are what are elicited by the doctor during examination and this is only part, and some would say a much lesser part, of the entire clinical evaluation. Few would disagree that much the more important part is the taking of a history, or if you like the elicitation of the patient's symptoms, which then necessarily leads to whatever type of examination and in whatever detail is subsequently required. As we saw in the lumbar disc hernia section, the diagnosis is made in the history section of the interview, when the patient *must* describe sciatica which means pain of a particular quality, quite different from the quality of low-back pain, and going below the knee. The subsequent physical examination indicates the severity of the clinical expression of the disc hernia and whether there is super-added nerve root dysfunction. The clinical examination, therefore, is in no way diagnostic of lumbar disc hernias or indeed of many other lumbar spine pathologies. Investigations including plain films and MRI scanning are even further remote from diagnosis with scans in particular there to confirm that a disc hernia is present on the side and at the level the surgeon suspects, when surgery is contemplated after an adequate non-operative treatment regimen has been completed and seen to fail.[11,12] With great respect to our general practitioner (GP) colleagues, who now have been granted free access to MRI scanning in our hospital, we hope that they will throw away their request cards and stick to good old-fashioned medical protocol and refer a patient with a suspected disc hernia, who is not doing well with physiotherapy or the passage of time to the spinal surgeon who can then evaluate the patient expertly and, of course, be in the most appropriate position to request scanning.[13] Not only is open access to scanning deleterious to the patient, but it is also deleterious to many other patients, often delaying the investigation of more serious pathologies. That patients are rushing in their hoards into the scanner to see what is wrong with them when patients who already have a clinical diagnosis of a significant disc hernia or even tumour have to wait for months is totally unacceptable and must represent an appalling waste of NHS time and money.

As Waddell has so succinctly stated[14] *there is considerable radiological concern about the overuse of these investigations (CT and MRI scanning) in non-specific low-back pain. However, investigation leads directly to treatment. These investigations should be ordered on clear clinical indications according to radiological guidelines.*[15]

Notwithstanding, and while extending the same care and courtesy to our medico-legal complainants as we do to our spinal patients, it has to be said that individuals with very inappropriate clinical histories combined with very inappropriate physical findings are commonly complainants and rarely clinic patients, and will not generally do well with surgery to the point where the wisdom of commissioning scans is open to considerable question.

In the early nineties Waddell[16] noted a 40% higher rate of back surgery in the US than any other country and more than

5 times that of the UK, and found that there was an almost linear relationship between back surgery rates and the per capita supply of orthopaedic and neurosurgeons in the country and such countries with high back surgery rates also had higher rates of other discretionary procedures, such as tonsillectomy and hysterectomy. These trends illustrated the large impact of health system differences on rates of back surgery and, of course, outcomes. Regrettably, the differences have now risen by an order of magnitude with the US having at least a 10 times higher rate of lumbar spine surgery and much greater than 10 times as regards lumbar spine fusion. Nachemson has particularly focused on the lumbar spine both as regards basic biological and biomechanical science but also as regards the epidemiology of back pain, and its response to surgery.

THE FAILURES OF SPINE SURGEONS

Prof. Nachemson[17] recently wrote a very critical account of the over-zealous performance of back surgery in a review article entitled "failed back surgery syndrome is syndrome of the failed back surgeon". He considered the subject under five headings which were the first, second, third, fourth and fifth failures of spine surgeons.

The five failures of spine surgeons

1. A lack of a scientific basis for the surgical indications for low-back pain
2. The relative absence of any scientific evidence of efficacy and effectiveness of our treatment methods
3. Willingness to be influenced by market forces of instrument manufacturers or well respected colleagues, who have invented a new implant
4. Inadequate reading of the literature on spinal fusion procedures performed primarily as well as repeat surgery
5. Disregard for the predictive value of psychosocial factors, particularly, with regard to repeat surgery

The first failure was that *it is generally agreed that there is a lack of scientific basis for the surgical indications for low-back pain alone*, i.e. low-back pain without sciatica or neurological sequelae. He went into detail about the low predictive value for low-back pain from spinal X-rays and there were always poorer results, when psychosocial factors in the work place or compensation prevail.

Like Nachemson, we are also very supportive of proposals made by Roland and van Tulder[18] (Table 8.2), who showed epidemiologically in meta-analytical reviews of the X-ray literature that there was no firm evidence supporting an association between ordinary X-ray findings, such as degeneration (whether slight or advanced), spondylosis, spondylolisthesis, transitional vertebra, Scheuermann's disease and non-specific back pain. Yet despite these findings patients are operated for these *conditions*, although no scientifically admissible evidence exists for a link between these X-ray findings and pain in any epidemiological sense.

Table 8.2   None of these is a risk factor for back pain (from Roland and van Tulder).

Slight degeneration	Almost half of patients with this finding on radiography do not have back pain, so this finding may not be related to the patient's pain
Advanced disc degeneration	Roughly 40% of patients with this finding do not have back pain, so this finding may be unrelated
Spondylosis	Roughly half of patients with this finding do not have back pain, so this finding may be unrelated
Spondylolisthesis	Roughly half of patients with this finding do not have back pain, so this finding may be unrelated
Spina bifida	Roughly half of patients with this finding do not have back pain, so this finding may be unrelated
Transitional vertebrae	Roughly half of patients with this finding do not have back pain, so this finding may be unrelated
Scheuermann's disease	More than 40% of patients with this finding do not have back pain, so this finding may be unrelated

In addition labelling patients with these poorly defined syndromes actually makes them worse.[19] Not surprisingly, there is little clinical validity in demonstrating a disc hernia on CT or MRI scanning.

The second failure of spine surgeons was *the relative absence of any scientific evidence of efficacy and effectiveness of our treatment methods.* We need this evidence but spine surgeons largely avoid attempts to find it. A recent Cochrane*[,20] review demonstrated categorically that disc surgery by ordinary laminotomy or by microdiscectomy was significantly better than enzyme injections (chemonucleolysis) both of which were significantly better than continued conservative care, while there was no evidence in favour of epidural steroids or bed rest. Nor was there any evidence for percutaneous or laser disc techniques, while on the contrary a few randomised controlled trials (RCTs) exist with negative results.[21] Of considerable interest is that on review of lumbar spine fusion for degenerative disc disease there was not one RCT comparing fusion surgery with any type of conservative or non-operative treatment![22].

The Cochrane Hierarchy

- Prospective RCT
- Prospective controlled trial
- Retrospective controlled trial
- Uncontrolled investigation
- Personal communication or what the boss says! – the lowest of the low!

It also demonstrated the serial reduction in success rates when the inventors' of the techniques first report is then followed by subsequent case series, prospective controlled trials and finally RCTs (Table 8.3). It is essential to do a valid study with concealed random allocation of patients to comparison groups and with few lost to follow-up. Thus, looking at The Cochrane Hierarchy we can see that the most rigorous investigation, the prospective RCT, would, say, for straight forward spinal fusion, randomly allocate patients to treatment and non-treatment groups of sufficient numbers predicted from what we call a

---

*Archie Cochrane, a famous British epidemiologist, pioneered the best possible experimental practice.

Table 8.3   Common evolution of new method/technology for treatment of low-back pain and sciatica.

	Per cent success		
	Percutaneous lumbar discectomy	Instrumented posterior fusion	Anterior metal cage fusion
Inventors first report	90	95	90
Subsequent case series	80	75	80
Prospective case control			
2-year follow-up	70	60	60
RCT, blinded unbiased			
2-year follow-up	40	40	?

power calculation to provide results of statistical significance. This would be a prospective study in that we would then after randomisation treat the patient group and the patients should be followed up for an adequate length of time, which for low-back pain a 5-year period might be considered a minimum (it has been shown that for simple disc hernias surgical benefit in terms of relief of sciatica is lost at about 4 years with treated patients now being no different from those treated non-surgically). Then, to reduce bias as much as possible the clinicians involved in management should not be those who assess the outcomes who in turn, if possible, should be blinded to whether a person belongs to the treatment or non-treatment groups. It is conventional to accept a better than 95% probability of the results being correct, and thus, if the study was repeated then the same results would be obtained on 19 out of 20 occasions.

Then comes the prospective controlled trial but not randomised, followed by the retrospective controlled trial, where we look back at a treatment group and compare it with an untreated group. Then, we get to the investigation with no controls at all and finally personal communication – "I've done a hundred of these operations and they were all successful" (a sort of claim that is not all that uncommon).

At a number of international meetings in 1998, orthopaedic surgeons were asked whether they would prescribe a fusion for chronic low-back pain and at the same time if they would be

Table 8.4 Orthopaedic surgeons' response in mentometer polls 1998. Would you send a chronic, idiopathic low-back patient to fusion surgery.

Country	Yes (%)	Would undergo fusion themselves (%)
USA	45	10
Great Britain	35	5
Sweden	30	7

prepared to undergo the procedure themselves. Table 8.4 shows the interesting but perhaps not unexpected result.

The third failure of spine surgeons is their *willingness to be influenced by market forces of instrument manufacturers or well respected colleagues who have invented a new implant for spine surgeons.* The several hundred % increase in the rate of lumbar fusion has occurred in all industrialised countries over the last decade with no scientific basis to it. Indeed, it would appear that Wall Street medical analysts actually believe that 40% of back pain patients need a fusion, thus, potentially driving merger frenzy amongst the instrument companies boosting their turnovers!

The fourth failure of spine surgeons concerns *adequate reading of the literature on spinal fusion procedures performed primarily as well as repeat surgery.* No study of fusion operations following scientific guidelines has shown better than 60% good or excellent results from primary fusion and around 30% for repeat surgery. The return to work in primary procedures was no more than 40% for anterior fusions and 16% following posterior fusions. Those with illness behaviour fared much worse.

The fifth and most important failure of spine surgeons was their *disregard for the predictive value of psychosocial factors particularly with regard to repeat surgery but also primary surgery,* and Nachemson pointed out exactly the same factors that Waddell and Main have done over the last two decades. He concluded with this statement: *"In this competitive world with a shrinking health care budget hip surgeons can point to impressive results of total hip replacements with proven economic benefits for society and excellent results in patients also in revision surgery. Spinal surgeons are far behind and unless this situation is corrected and efficacy and effectiveness are proven there is a danger that they may be left out in the cold".*

Surgeons do indeed have an enthusiastic approach to their chosen art and are very often extremely skilled in the performance of operations that can be technically very difficult. This may seem a very important prerogative but of greater importance is the essential algorithm or protocol leading up to surgery – *the what, the why and the when.* What operation is optimal as a surgical solution for a particular problem; what is the optimal timing of such a procedure; why is a surgical solution being sought when other therapeutic avenues may be addressed? These are fundamentally crucial decisions on the way to "how" (the procedure is performed). The skill of the surgeon only becomes relevant if the previous questions have been satisfied. As regards lumbar spine surgery the knife can be a very satisfactory outcome for both patient and surgeon but perhaps the surgeon can do some self-administered psychosocial testing by sitting down, taking stock of the situation, and asking himself if it really is in the patient's best interest to be treated by a man in a white coat with a scalpel in his pocket. Indeed, unless we all address that question and do so with a considerable degree of urgency, we shall, as Nachemson foresees, be rapidly left out in the cold.

Despite greater knowledge and expertise in health care resources, chronic disability resulting from non-specific low-back pain is rising exponentially in the western world.[23] Not only has medical care not solved the problem of low-back pain but may indeed be reinforcing and exacerbating the problem as Waddell has described. Indeed, some of the disabling pain syndromes that we are dealing with today are actually *nomogenic diseases* – they are diseases created by lawyers or by politicians, while we may well say that the failed back syndrome is an *iatrogenic disease* created by surgeons. The numbers of millions of days per annum lost due to chronic low-back disability has risen by more than an order of magnitude from about 10 million days per annum lost in the mid-fifties to more than 105 million in the early nineties and probably approaching 200 million days per annum lost at this millennium. Non-specific low-back pain (simple backache) is commonly related to physical strain, although, as already pointed out, these are often normal daily activities and perhaps, in reality, it usually develops spontaneously. Non-specific low-back pain may be very painful and often spreads as referred pain to one or both buttocks or thighs but it should be a benign self-limiting condition. Epidemiological studies have shown that simple backache has a point prevalence of approximately 15–30%, a 1-month prevalence of 30–40% and a lifetime prevalence of 60–80%. In other words about one in five of the adult population will have back pain at any given moment, a third will have an episode of back pain during the course of a month and three quarters will admit to having an episode of back pain during their adult life. There is no evidence that the prevalence of low-back pain is lower in the US than in Europe and there is no historical evidence that low-back pain is any different, any more common or any more severe than it always has been.

In the mid-1980s, Nachemson was asked by the Swedish government to review the state of play about back pain because the government were finding it very expensive for the welfare state. He found that in the early 1970s, 1% of working people in Sweden that were insured had been absent from work due to back pain and this increased to 8% in 1987. Moreover patients were off work for longer, 20 days going up to 34 days per year. In the late 1980s, Sweden set the world record with an increase by 6% of individuals on permanent disability due to back problems from 1950 to 1990. About 650,000 Swedish workers are currently disabled due to non-specific pain disorders claiming to be work related and about 70% of these have unspecified back pain.

We have already seen that genetic factors are much more important than anything else in the development of disc degeneration and herniation as well as symptoms therefrom, but the Finnish identical twin cohort study also showed that in the bottom two spinal joints, where most back symptoms are thought to arise, only 1.5% of back pain could be linked to the subjects workloads or to their recreational activities in a biomechanical sense. Most was genetic but a large proportion, of the order of 40%, was inexplicable but not mechanical. This was why they concluded that mechanical factors do not seem to induce disc changes. Another study[24] compared 46 patients operated on for sciatica due to a disc hernia with 46 age and sex matched controls performing the same type of work but who had never had sciatica and never had back pain. These controls volunteered to have MRI scans of the lumbar spine. Psychosocial factors and work perception factors in both patients in controls were also studied. No less than three-quarters of the normal group exhibited disc hernias on MRI scanning but there were two important differences between the groups. The operated group was psychosocially much more disturbed and the disc hernia was located more laterally interfering with the local nerve root.

> ### Boos
>
> *"There is, therefore, little support for informing a patient with back pain and some leg pain in whom a disc hernia has been diagnosed that this is work related as such findings occur without pain in an astonishing 76% of the population".*

In addition, as we have seen, labelling patients makes them ill. That is why we have to find another way of explaining to patients why they have their pain and there is no earthly reason why we cannot be honest and say we simply do not know, at least on balance.

In addition, epidemiological studies have shown that strong muscles[25] neither protect from back pain nor has spinal mobility any predictive value. Certain types of lift and working positions should be avoided and, in particular, twisting lifts. Thus, some association appears to exist between load and severe symptoms. There is, however, no evidence that structural damage and, in particular, disc pathology is any way affected. Certainly, a sudden significant twisting lift would be regarded as a more discrete *injury* rather than generating non-specific low-back pain. This is supported by evidence that work place inspections and the institution of safer lifting methods reduce the number of objective injuries but not of the non-specific low-back pain episodes.[23] It has also been shown repeatedly that workers insurance compensation significantly increases the number of objective injuries but much more so the absence rate for non-specific back pain.[23] Again, there have been significant correlations published between increasing absence or work disability with increased take home pay.

> ## Canadian study
>
> 5000 uninsured patients versus 6000 insured patients
>
> Question – how did the back pain occur?
>
> Answer – Uninsured, 33% work related
>   Insured, 90% work related

This Canadian study of all of 11,000 individuals carries very much more weight than studies of smaller numbers.

Clearly, we all react to economic incentives but the results of surgery are significantly different between patients and complainants, the latter always doing worse in all published series. Nachemson points out that this applies not only to back surgery but also to shoulder tendon repair (return to work 42% in compensation cases and 94% in non-compensation cases); carpal tunnel release (12 weeks to return to work in workers' compensation versus 3 weeks for non-workers' compensation); inguinal hernia repair (111 days in compensation cases versus 34 days in non-compensation cases). The same can be said for head injury in that compensation prolongs symptoms and disability despite the head injury presenting no objective neurological findings. We are perhaps making people sicker by our insurance schemes.

Job satisfaction and the work environment are very important factors, particularly, for back pain with job satisfaction being the strongest independent variable for disability.[27] In one comparative study between 60 healthy controls, 60 patients with a 6-week absence from work and 60 patients with a 3-month absence from work a physiotherapist and a physician looked at the work places and found no difference in workload.[28] However, the work environment and work satisfaction were very significantly worse in the symptomatic patients.

Another study looked at 3000 blue collar workers in the Boeing aircraft factory following them for 4 years and measuring a host of psychological and psychosocial variables as well as ergonomic and biomechanical ones.[26] Two hundred and fifty workers were off for 1 day or more due to back pain but workload, muscle strength, fitness, mobility, sex and age were not significant factors in this regard. *Significant factors were the past history of back trouble, smoking and psychosocial factors. The simple question "do you like what you are doing, do you like your fellow worker, do you like your foreman?" with a response of "no" demonstrated a significantly increased risk of disabling back pain within the next year.*

Boeing study

3000 workers, 250 absent 1 day or more

Workload, muscle strength, fitness, mobility, sex and age not significant factors

Past history of back trouble, smoking and psychosocial factors significant

A similar study was carried out looking at nurse aids and Volvo workers evaluating how much they bent and lifted every day and at the end of the day they were asked if this was a heavy day for your back which they then graded.[29] The good day or bad day for the back had nothing to do with the amount of lifting or bending these nurses and workers actually did. Rather, it had to do in the nurse aids with disturbances at work and for the factory workers it was correlated with stress, which could be corroborated by measurements of urinary levels of stress hormones. *Thus, mental stress and irritation are much more important than biomechanical loading and this is supported by many other studies.* As these psychosocial work factors are so important the International Association for the Study of Pain has recently proposed that *back disability should be work related for perhaps the first 6–8 weeks after which it becomes psychological back pain and should not be looked upon or reimbursed as a work-related disease.* This view is based on the biological findings that whatever injury there is it should have healed within approximately 6 weeks.[30] Clearly, this does not apply to injuries with major structural damage but then few individuals have. Even when objective injury is demonstrable, disability has much to do with motivation and work enjoyment. Swedish air force pilots, who had ejected from aircraft and sustained burst fractures, were all back to work within a few months.

In this country, the Confederation of British Industry estimates that back pain costs £208.00 for every employee each year and that at any one time 430,000 people in the UK are receiving various social security benefits primarily for back pain. As this disability from back pain in people of working age is one of the most dramatic failures of healthcare in recent years, and has a great impact on the lives of those affected and their families as well as a major effect on industry through absenteeism and avoidable costs, the Faculty of Occupational Medicine carried out a detailed review of this matter and produced guidelines providing a new approach to back-pain management at work based on the best available scientific evidence and made practical recommendations on how to tackle the occupational health aspects of this problem.[31] There were 18 members of the Faculty Working Group representing occupational physicians, nurses, GPs, the Departments of Health, Social Security and the Health and Safety Executive, Economists and the Orthopaedic Surgeon was Gordon Waddell. This review should really be compulsory reading for anybody involved in the management of low-back pain. The guidelines consist of *recommendations* accompanied by *evidence statements* with ratings of the strength of that evidence. For instance, *** represents strong evidence (consistent findings in multiple high quality scientific studies); ** moderate evidence (consistent findings in fewer, smaller or lower quality scientific studies); * limited or contradictory evidence (one scientific study or inconsistent findings in multiple scientific studies) and no scientific evidence. They point out that while non-specific low-back pain can be occupational in the sense that it is common in adults of working age, frequently affects capacity for work, and often presents for occupational health care, it is commonly assumed that this means that low-back pain is caused by work but the relationship between the physical demands of work and low-back pain is complex and inconsistent.

A clear distinction should be made between the presence of symptoms, the reporting of low-back pain, attributing symptoms to work, reporting "injury", seeking health care, loss of time from work and long term damage. Low-back pain in the occupational setting must be seen against the high background prevalence in recurrence rates of low-back symptoms and to a lesser extent disability in the adult population. Workers in heavy manual jobs do report rather more low-back symptoms, but most people in lighter jobs or even those who are not working have similar symptoms. Jobs with greater

Table 18.5

***Most adults (60–80%) experience low-back pain at some time and it is often persistent or recurrent.

***Physical demands of work (manual materials handling, lifting, bending, twisting and whole body vibration) are a risk factor for the incidence (onset) of low-back pain, but overall it appears that the size of the effect is less than that of other individual, non-occupational and unidentified factors.

***Care seeking and disability due to low-back pain depend more on complex individual and work-related psychosocial factors than on clinical features or physical demands of work.

***The single most consistent predictor of future low-back pain and work loss is a previous history of low-back pain.

***X-ray and MRI findings have no predictive value for future low-back pain or disability.

***Back-function testing machines have no predictive value for future low-back pain or disability.

***For symptom-free people, individual psychosocial findings are a risk factor for the incidence (onset) of low-back pain but overall the size of the effect is small.

***In patients with non-specific low-back pain X-ray and MRI findings do not correlate with clinical symptoms or work capacity.

***Advice to continue ordinary activities of living as normally as possible despite the pain can give equivalent or faster symptomatic recovery than traditional medical treatment.

***Most workers with low-back pain are able to continue working or to return to work within a few days or weeks, even if they still have some residual or recurrent symptoms and they do not need to wait till they are completely pain free.

***Most clinical interventions are quite ineffective at returning people to work once they have been off work for a protracted period with low-back pain.

***The longer a worker is off work with low-back pain the lower their chances of ever returning to work. Off work 4–12 weeks they have a 10–40% risk of still being off work at 1 year and after 1–2 years absence it is unlikely they will return to any form of work.

physical demands commonly have a higher rate of reported low-back injuries, but most of these "injuries" are related to normal everyday activities, such as bending and lifting. There is usually little if any objective evidence of tissue damage and the relationship between job demands and symptoms or injury rates is inconsistent. Physical stresses may overload certain structures in individual cases but, in general, there is little evidence that physical loading in modern work causes permanent damage. They summarise this background as follows: "*physical demands of work can precipitate individual attacks of low-back pain, certain individuals may be more susceptible and certain jobs may be higher risk but, viewed overall, physical demands of work only account for a modest proportion of the total impact of low-back pain occurring in workers.*"

The Group looked at 173 publications including the ones already referred to in this chapter. Some of the more important *** (strong evidence) pieces of evidence leading to important recommendations are shown in Table 18.5.

Individual and work-related psychosocial factors play an important role in persisting symptoms and disability and workers' own beliefs that their low-back pain was caused by their work and their own expectations about inability to return to work are particularly important.

One controlled trial[32] demonstrated that ergonomic teaching was far less effective in reducing absence due to back pain than personal contact and apparently low-back disability was reduced by 70% by a firm employing a special nurse, who called her employees and said *you are a vital part of our staff, your work is important and your job is waiting for you, could we help you to come back.*

REFERENCES

1. Foy M, Fagg P (Eds). Medicolegal reporting in orthopaedic trauma, Third edition. 2002.
2. Pilowsky J. Abnormal illness behaviour. British Journal of Medical Psychology 1969, 42: 347–351.
3. Waddell G, Kummel EG, Lotto WN, Graham JD, Hall H, McCullough JA. Failed lumbar disc surgery and repeat surgery following industrial injuries. Journal of Bone and Joint Surgery 1979, 61A: 201–207.
4. Waddell G, McCullough JA, Kummel EG, Venner RM. Non-organic physical signs in low back pain. Spine 1980, 5: 117–125.

5. Waddell G, Bircher M, Finlayson D, Main CJ. Symptoms and signs: physical disease or illness behavior? Table 1. British Medical Journal 1984, 289: 740.

6. Waddell G, Main CJ, Morris EW, Di Paola MP, Gray ICM. Chronic low back pain, psychological distress and illness behaviour. Spine 1984, 9: 209–213.

7. Waddell G, Morris EW, Di Paola MP, Bircher M, Finlayson D. A concept of illness tested as an improved basis for surgical decisions in low-back disorders. Spine 1986, 11: 712–719.

8. Waddell G, Riley S, Torsney B, Allan DB, Morris EW, Di Paola MP, Bircher M, Finlayson D. Assessment of the outcome of low back surgery. Journal of Bone and Joint Surgery 1988, 70B: 723–727.

9. Main CJ, Wood PLR, Hollis S, Spanswick CC, Waddell G. The distress and risk assessment method. A simple patient classification to identify distress and evaluate the risk of poor outcome. Spine 1992, 17: 42–51.

10. Main CJ, Waddell G. Behavioural responses to examination. A reappraisal of the interpretation of "non-organic signs". Spine 1998; 23: 2367–2371.

11. Nachemson AL. Editorial – Lumbar disc disease. Current Orthopaedics 1995, 9: 11–72.

12. Dickson RA, Butt WP. Mini-symposium: lumbar disc disease. (i) Clinical and radiological assessment. Current Orthopaedics 1995, 9: 73–84.

13. Butt WP. Editorials. Magnetic resonance imaging of the spine. British Journal of Rheumatology 1994, 33: 793–797.

14. Waddell G. Low back pain: a twentieth century health care enigma. Spine 1996, 21: 2820–2825.

15. Royal College of Radiologists. Making the best use of a Department of Clinical Radiology: guidelines for doctors, Third edition. RCR, London. 1995, pp. 1–96.

16. Cherkin DC, Deyo RA, Loeser JD, Bush T, Waddell G. An international comparison of back surgery rates. Spine 1994, 19: 1201–1206.

17. Nachemson AL. Failed back surgery syndrome is syn-drome of failed back surgeons. The Pain Clinic 1999, 11: 271–284.

18. Roland M, van Tulder MW. Should radiologists change the way they report plain radiography of the spine. Viewpoint. Lancet 1998, 352: 229–230.

19. Abenhaim L, Rossignol M, Gobeille D, Bonvalot Y, Fines P, Scott S. The prognostic consequences in the making of the initial medical diagnosis of work-related back injuries. Spine 1995, 20(7): 791–795.

20. Gibson JNA, Waddell G. The management of lumbar disc prolapse (protocol for a Cochrane Review). In Cochrane Library, Issue 4. 1998, Update software, Oxford.

21. Chatterjee S, Foy PM, Findlay GF. Report of a control clinical trial comparing automated percutaneous lumbar discectomy and microdiscectomy in the treatment of contained lumbar disc herniation. Spine 1995, 20: 734–738.

22. Gibson JNR, Waddell G. The surgical treatment of degenerative lumbar spondylosis. (Protocol for a Cochrane Review). In Cochrane Library, Issue 4. 1998, Update Software, Oxford.

23. Nachemson AL. Back pain: delimiting the problem in the next millennium. International Journal of Law and Psychiatry 1999, 22: 473–490.

24. Boos N, Rieder R, Schade V, Spratt KF, Semmer N, Aebi M. The diagnostic accuracy of magnetic resonance imaging, work perception and psychosocial factors in identifying symptomatic disc herniations. Spine 1995, 20: 2613–2615.

25. Bigos S, Battie MC, Spengler DM, Fisher LD, Fordyce WE, Hansson TH, Nachemson AL, Wortley MD. A prospective study of work perceptions

and psychosocial factors affecting the report of back injury. Spine 1991,1: 1–16.

26. Hall H. Personal communication with AL Nachemson, Toronto. 1996.
27. Bergenhudd H, Nilsson B. Back pain in middle age; occupational workload and psychologic factors an epidemiologic survey. Spine 1988, 13: 58–60.
28. Vällfors B. Acute, subacute and chronic low back pain. Scandinavian Journal of Rehabilitation Medicine 1985 Suppl 11: 1–98.
29. Lundberg U, Granqvist M, Hansson T *et al*. Psychological and physiological stress responses during repetitive work at an assembly line. Work Stress 1989, 3: 143–153.
30. Fordyce WE. Task force on pain in the workplace. In Back pain in the workplace. Management of disability and non-specific conditions. 1995, IASP Press, Seattle.
31. Carter JT, Birrell LN (Eds). Occupational health guidelines for the management of low back pain at work – principal recommendations. 2000, Faculty of Occupational Medicine, London.
32. Wood DJ. Design and evaluation of a back injury prevention program within a geriatric hospital. Spine 1987, 12: 77–82.

INDEX

Note: 'f' after a page number indicates a reference to a figure, 't' indicates a reference to a table.